Clinical Pathology for the Equine Practitioner

Editors

SALLYANNE L. DENOTTA
TRACY STOKOL

VETERINARY CLINICS OF NORTH AMERICA: EQUINE PRACTICE

www.vetequine.theclinics.com

Consulting Editor
THOMAS J. DIVERS

April 2020 • Volume 36 • Number 1

ELSEVIER

1600 John F. Kennedy Boulevard • Suite 1800 • Philadelphia, Pennsylvania, 19103-2899

http://www.vetequine.theclinics.com

VETERINARY CLINICS OF NORTH AMERICA: EQUINE PRACTICE Volume 36, Number 1
April 2020 ISSN 0749-0739, ISBN-13: 978-0-323-71277-4

Editor: Colleen Dietzler
Developmental Editor: Donald Mumford

Veterinary Clinics of North America: Equine Practice (ISSN 0749-0739) is published in April, August, and December by Elsevier Inc., 360 Park Avenue South, New York, NY 10010-1710. Business and Editorial Offices: 1600 John F. Kennedy Blvd., Suite 1800, Philadelphia, PA 19103-2899. Subscription prices are $290.00 per year (domestic individuals), $585.00 per year (domestic institutions), $100.00 per year (domestic students/residents), $334.00 per year (Canadian individuals), $737.00 per year (Canadian institutions), $365.00 per year (international individuals), $737.00 per year (international institutions), $100.00 per year (Canadian students/residents), and $180.00 per year (international students/residents). To receive student/resident rate, orders must be accompanied by name of affiliated institution, date of term, and the signature of program/residency coordinator on institution letterhead. Orders will be billed at individual rate until proof of status is received. Foreign air speed delivery is included in all *Clinics* subscription prices. All prices are subject to change without notice. **POSTMASTER:** Send address changes to *Veterinary Clinics of North America: Equine Practice*, 3251 Riverport Lane, Maryland Heights, MO 63043. Customer Service (orders, claims, online, change of address): Elsevier Health Sciences Division, Subscription **Customer Service, 3251 Riverport Lane, Maryland Heights, MO 63043. Tel: 1-800-654-2452 (U.S. and Canada); 314-447-8871 (outside U.S. and Canada). Fax: 314-447-8029. E-mail: journalscustomerservice-usa@elsevier.com (for print support);** E-mail: **journalsonlinesupport-usa@elsevier.com (for online support).**

Reprints. For copies of 100 or more of articles in this publication, please contact the Commercial Reprints Department, Elsevier Inc., 360 Park Avenue South, New York, NY 10010-1710. Tel.: 212-633-3874; Fax: 212-633-3820; E-mail: reprints@elsevier.com.

Veterinary Clinics of North America: Equine Practice is covered in *MEDLINE/PubMed (Index Medicus), Excerpta Medica, Current Contents/Agriculture, Biology and Environmental Sciences,* and *ISI.*

Contributors

CONSULTING EDITOR

THOMAS J. DIVERS, DVM
Diplomate, American College of Veterinary Internal Medicine; Diplomate, American College of Veterinary Emergency and Critical Care; Steffen Professor of Veterinary Medicine, Department of Clinical Sciences, Section of Large Animal Medicine, Cornell University College of Veterinary Medicine, Ithaca, New York, USA

EDITORS

SALLYANNE L. DENOTTA, DVM, PhD
Diplomate, American College of Veterinary Internal Medicine; Clinical Assistant Professor, Large Animal Clinical Sciences, College of Veterinary Medicine, University of Florida, Gainesville, Florida, USA

TRACY STOKOL, BVSc, PhD
Diplomate, American College of Veterinary Pathologists (Clinical Pathology); Professor, Department of Population Medicine and Diagnostic Sciences, Cornell University College of Veterinary Medicine, Ithaca, New York, USA

AUTHORS

MICHELLE HENRY BARTON, DVM, PhD
Diplomate of the American College of Veterinary Internal Medicine, Large Animal Internal Medicine; Director of Clinical Academic Affairs, Fuller E. Callaway Endowed Professor, Josiah Meigs Distinguished Teaching Professor, Department of Large Animal Medicine, College of Veterinary Medicine, University of Georgia, Athens, Georgia, USA

DOROTHEE BIENZLE, DVM, PhD
Diplomate, American College of Veterinary Pathologists; Professor, Department of Pathobiology, University of Guelph, Guelph, Ontario, Canada

RANA BOZORGMANESH, BVetMed
Diplomate, American College of Veterinary Internal Medicine; Associate Internist, Hagyard Equine Medical Institute, McGee Medical Center, Lexington, Kentucky, USA

MARJORY B. BROOKS, DVM
Diplomate, American College of Veterinary Internal Medicine; Director, Comparative Coagulation Laboratory, Animal Health Diagnostic Center, Cornell University, Ithaca, New York, USA

NIMET BROWNE, DVM, MPH
Diplomate, American College of Veterinary Internal Medicine; Associate
Internist, Hagyard Equine Medical Institute, McGee Medical Center, Lexington,
Kentucky, USA

LAURENT L. COUETIL, DVM, PhD
Diplomate, American College of Veterinary Internal Medicine - Large Animal Internal
Medicine; Professor of Large Animal Medicine, Department of Veterinary Clinical
Sciences, Purdue University College of Veterinary Medicine, West Lafayette, Indiana,
USA

SALLYANNE L. DENOTTA, DVM, PhD
Diplomate, American College of Veterinary Internal Medicine; Clinical Assistant Professor,
Large Animal Clinical Sciences, College of Veterinary Medicine, University of Florida,
Gainesville, Florida, USA

THOMAS J. DIVERS, DVM
Diplomate, American College of Veterinary Internal Medicine; Diplomate, American
College of Veterinary Emergency and Critical Care; Steffen Professor of Veterinary
Medicine, Department of Clinical Sciences, Section of Large Animal Medicine, Cornell
University College of Veterinary Medicine, Ithaca, New York, USA

MELISSA M. ESSER, DVM, MS
Diplomate, American College of Veterinary Internal Medicine; Assistant
Professor, Department of Large Animal Clinical Sciences, Veterinary Medical
Center, College of Veterinary Medicine, Michigan State University, East Lansing,
Michigan, USA

KELSEY A. HART, DVM, PhD
Diplomate of the American College of Veterinary Internal Medicine, Large Animal Internal
Medicine; Director of the Veterinary Medical Scientist Training Program, Associate
Professor, Department of Large Animal Medicine, College of Veterinary Medicine,
University of Georgia, Athens, Georgia, USA

SAMUEL D.A. HURCOMBE, BSc, BVMS, MS
Diplomate, American College of Veterinary Internal Medicine; Diplomate, American
College of Veterinary Emergency and Critical Care; Associate Professor Emergency and
Critical Care, New Bolton Center, School of Veterinary Medicine, University of
Pennsylvania, Kennett Square, Pennsylvania, USA

ALICIA LONG, DVM
Resident, Department of Clinical Studies, New Bolton Center, Kennett Square,
Pennsylvania, USA

ASHLEIGH W. NEWMAN, VMD
Diplomate, American College of Veterinary Pathologists (Clinical Pathology); Assistant
Clinical Professor, Department of Population Medicine and Diagnostic Sciences, Cornell
University College of Veterinary Medicine, Ithaca, New York, USA

ROSE NOLEN-WALSTON, DVM
Diplomate, American College of Veterinary Internal Medicine; Associate Professor,
Department of Clinical Studies, New Bolton Center, Kennett Square, Pennsylvania,
USA

HAROLD C. SCHOTT II, DVM, PhD
Diplomate, American College of Veterinary Internal Medicine; Professor, Department of Large Animal Clinical Sciences, Veterinary Medical Center, College of Veterinary Medicine, Michigan State University, East Lansing, Michigan, USA

NATHAN M. SLOVIS, DVM, CHT
Diplomate, American College of Veterinary Internal Medicine; Hagyard Equine Medical Institute, Director, McGee Medical Center, Lexington, Kentucky, USA

TRACY STOKOL, BVSc, PhD
Diplomate, American College of Veterinary Pathologists (Clinical Pathology); Professor, Department of Population Medicine and Diagnostic Sciences, Cornell University College of Veterinary Medicine, Ithaca, New York, USA

CRAIG A. THOMPSON, DVM
Diplomate, American College of Veterinary Pathology; Clinical Associate Professor of Clinical Pathology, Department of Comparative Pathobiology, Purdue University College of Veterinary Medicine, West Lafayette, Indiana, USA

Contents

Clinical pathology results are only as good as the quality of samples and accompanying information submitted to the diagnostic laboratory. The frustration of nondiagnostic or equivocal test results can often be avoided by taking the time to follow sample handling and submission guidelines. This article discusses preanalytical errors that commonly affect the accuracy of hematology, chemistry, and cytology testing, and offers practical tips for preventing these errors and maximizing diagnostic yield.

This article uses a case-based approach, complemented with diagnostic algorithms and images, to highlight hematologic changes of pathologic relevance in horses, namely, marked erythrocytosis, anemia or leukocytosis, inflammatory leukograms, lymphocytosis in adult horses, thrombocytopenia, and pancytopenia. These hematologic abnormalities occur with certain diseases and their identification can help clinicians narrow down differential diagnostic lists. This article highlights the importance of blood smear examination, particularly, but not only, when numerical red flags are identified on automated blood counts.

This article describes the indications for sampling of bone marrow, the technical aspects of obtaining marrow core biopsies and aspirates, and the preparation of marrow smears. All aspects are illustrated with clinical cases. The information that can be expected from the pathologist's report of marrow samples is outlined, and the clinical features and prognosis of different types of leukemia are detailed.

Horses with clinical signs of unprovoked or excessive hemorrhage should be evaluated for underlying platelet defects or coagulopathies. This article provides an overview of preliminary screening and definitive tests to assess coagulation and identify hemostatic defects in horses, as well as a review of the hemostatic disorders most frequently encountered in clinical practice.

The assessment of blood analytes in racehorses can provide useful data on performance and health. The horses' adaptive responses to training that occur to optimize performance should be considered when interpreting alterations seen in laboratory results. Similarly, the alterations observed in laboratory test results can identify subclinical and clinical disease and be helpful for identifying organ dysfunction and, in many cases, monitoring progress and response to treatment. This article discusses hematologic and biochemical tests that are important in the evaluation of performance and health in racehorses.

Serum amyloid A (SAA) is a marker of inflammation and infection in the horse that can be assessed in the field, with rapid and marked changes following initiation of an inflammatory stimulus. This quality of SAA also makes its clinical use challenging, because even small inflammatory conditions can cause large changes in SAA concentrations. Review of the current literature provides guidelines regarding the documented responses of SAA to various conditions, which can be applied to specific clinical cases. The practitioner is encouraged to use SAA in conjunction with physical examination and other diagnostic modalities to guide treatment and monitor case progression.

Point-of-care testing (POCT) refers to benchtop diagnostic modalities that have been translated into portable and easy-to-use formats suitable for patient-side use. Recent advances in diagnostic technology have allowed the development of a growing collection of POCT assays available to equine practitioners. Advantages include rapid results that reduce initial guesswork and promote diagnosis-targeted patient care, which may ultimately provide better clinical outcomes. Small handheld devices comprise most POCT technologies, providing qualitative or quantitative determination of an increasing range of analytes, including critical care analyzers and, more recently, hematology and immunology analyzers. This article discusses commercially available equine POCT.

VETERINARY CLINICS OF NORTH AMERICA: EQUINE PRACTICE

RELATED SERIES

Veterinary Clinics of North America: Food Animal Practice

Preface

A Word of Thanks from the Editors

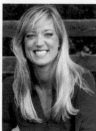   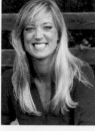

SallyAnne L. DeNotta, DVM, PhD   Tracy Stokol BVSc, PhD
Editors

Clinical pathology is an integral component of veterinary medicine, and we hope this issue of *Veterinary Clinics of North America: Equine Practice* will serve as a source of valuable and practical information for our equine veterinarian friends, colleagues, and equine-oriented students and trainees. We would like to thank Dr Tom Divers, as well as Don Mumford and Colleen Dietzler at Elsevier, for the opportunity to serve as coeditors of this issue. Most importantly, this project would not have been possible without our contributing authors, and for their time, expertise, and tremendous effort, we are so grateful.

—Sally and Tracy

SallyAnne L. DeNotta, DVM, PhD
Large Animal Clinical Sciences
College of Veterinary Medicine
University of Florida
PO Box 100136
Gainesville, FL 32610-0136, USA

Tracy Stokol, BVSc, PhD
Department of Population Medicine and
Diagnostic Sciences
College of Veterinary Medicine
Cornell University
S1-058 Schurman Hall
Upper Tower Road
Ithaca, NY, 14853-6401, USA

E-mail addresses:
s.denotta@ufl.edu (S.L. DeNotta)
ts23@cornell.edu (T. Stokol)

Vet Clin Equine 36 (2020) xi
https://doi.org/10.1016/j.cveq.2020.01.001
0749-0739/20/© 2020 Published by Elsevier Inc.

Practical Tips on Sample Handling for Hematology, Chemistry, and Cytology Testing for Equine Patients:
Getting More Bang for your Buck

Ashleigh W. Newman, VMD

KEYWORDS

- Clinical pathology • Error • Artifact • Equine • CBC • Sample handling
- Biochemistry

KEY POINTS

- Hematology: always submit a blood smear made at the time of sample collection to prevent in vitro sample aging from affecting cell morphologic evaluation.
- Chemistry
  - Promptly separate serum or heparinized plasma from cells.
  - Do not collect samples into or expose chemistry samples to EDTA.
- Cytology
  - Provide a detailed description of the sampled site and a succinct history.
  - For body fluids, submit a direct smear prepared at the time of collection and the fluid in an EDTA tube.
- Ship samples cool and overnight to avoid prolonged sample storage and in vitro aging artifacts.
- Do not expose hematologic or cytologic slides to formalin fumes.

INTRODUCTION

Veterinarians use clinical pathology testing to verify health on wellness visits or before elective surgeries, investigate physical examination abnormalities and clinical signs of disease, and monitor animals undergoing treatment or recovering from illness. Hematologic, biochemical, and cytologic testing are the most common diagnostic tests submitted by equine veterinarians for these purposes. Each of these areas has the potential to be affected by preanalytical errors, which are largely preventable.

Department of Population Medicine and Diagnostic Sciences, Cornell University College of Veterinary Medicine, S1-056 Schurman Hall, 602 Tower Road, Ithaca, NY 14853, USA
E-mail address: alw43@cornell.edu

Vet Clin Equine 36 (2020) 1–14
https://doi.org/10.1016/j.cveq.2019.12.002
0749-0739/20/© 2019 Elsevier Inc. All rights reserved.

Preanalytical errors include errors occurring before the actual testing of the sample, such as during sample collection (eg, selection of proper tube, separation of plasma or serum from cells for biochemical testing) and submission (eg, storage and shipping conditions).

Many preanalytical errors are related to prolonged in vitro sample storage, which can be minimized by overnight shipping samples to the testing laboratory. The extra cost is well worth it, when compared to trying to interpret or explain nondiagnostic or equivocal results to a client. The type of specimen (eg, whole blood, serum, plasma, joint fluid) and patient name should always be clearly written on the specimen label and request form.[1,2] The accompanying request form should include the owner name, animal identification, signalment, date of sample collection, veterinarian name, clinic's name, and contact information.[1,2] Often forgotten, but equally as important, particularly for cytology testing, is providing a succinct clinical history.

The famous saying "garbage in, garbage out" certainly applies to sample handling in clinical pathology. The objective of this article is to highlight common preanalytical errors and to start you off on the right foot with tips on how to submit high-quality samples for clinical pathology testing.

HEMATOLOGY

Hematologic testing refers to a hemogram or complete blood count (CBC), which provides both quantitative and qualitative data on red blood cells (RBCs), white blood cells (WBCs), and platelets. Total protein concentration as determined by refractometry, visual evaluation of plasma (ie, for hemolysis, icterus, and lipemia), and a crude measurement of fibrinogen concentration by heat precipitation are also provided by some laboratories. To accurately count cells, the sample must be collected into an anticoagulant, with ethylenediamine tetraacetic acid (EDTA, purple top tube) being the anticoagulant of choice.[3] On receipt in the laboratory, samples are grossly evaluated for macroclots. If present, these samples are canceled, as they inevitably produce erroneous results and the degree of inaccuracy cannot be predicted.[1,3] Clotting can be minimized by clean venipuncture using vacutainers or promptly transferring the collected blood from a syringe into the EDTA tube, followed by gently inverting the tube (about 3–4 times), to ensure thorough mixing of the blood with the anticoagulant. Blood samples should be refrigerated/kept cool if sample processing will be more than a few hours.[3] If mailing, the sample should be shipped with a cool pack but not in direct contact with ice.

White Blood Cells

Although an automated CBC can provide a reasonably accurate leukocyte differential for neutrophils, lymphocytes, and eosinophils on a fresh blood sample, examination of a blood smear provides additional useful information including the presence and degree of a left shift, toxic change, and infectious agents (see Tracy Stokol's article, "Hematology Red Flags: The Value of Blood Smear Examination in Horses," in this issue). A left shift is the presence of immature neutrophils, typically band neutrophils with rare earlier precursors (eg, metamyelocytes, myelocytes). Toxic change is characterized by cytoplasmic changes in neutrophils including increased basophilia, frothy vacuolization, and/or Döhle bodies. A left shift with or without toxic change indicates an inflammatory leukogram. The ability to detect these abnormalities, particularly a left shift, is hindered by prolonged sample storage. With storage, neutrophil nuclei swell, making it difficult to distinguish aged segmented neutrophils from true band neutrophils (**Fig. 1**).[3] "Pseudo-Döhle" bodies

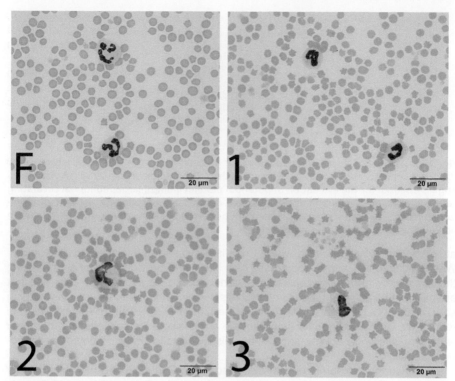

Fig. 1. Blood smears prepared from the same tube of EDTA-anticoagulated blood from a healthy horse. (*F*): Fresh blood smear made on the day of collection showing crisply segmented nuclei of neutrophils, (1) after one, (2) two, and (3) three days of storage at 4°C (refrigerated). The neutrophils display progressively increased nuclear swelling. Note the increased echinocyte formation and platelet clumping on day 3 (Wright stain). These changes would be exacerbated with the sample left at room temperature.

also form with sample aging, which can mimic toxic change. This dilemma can be avoided by providing a good-quality blood smear made at the time of sample collection, along with the EDTA blood. A good smear is made from about a 5 mm drop of blood and has a curved feathered edge that is approximately three-fourths along the slide to allow complete staining with automatic stainers (**Fig. 2**). A feathered edge is examined for platelet clumps, larger cells (eg, histiocytes, blasts), and infectious agents. Using too large a drop of blood results in excessively thick smears that may extend the length of the slide and lack a feathered edge. Blood smears should be rapidly air dried (eg, with a hairdryer directed to the back of the slide, particularly in hot, humid conditions) and kept at room temperature, with no need for heat fixing. If an initial evaluation is desired, one smear can be stained with rapid stains, for example, Diff-Quik, first. However, additional blood smears should be made, as submission of unstained smears is optimal to allow diagnostic laboratories use their preferred stain. Blood smears should be protected from condensation during shipping.[1]

In the absence of a fresh blood smear or knowledge of sample collection date (if not provided on the request form), an experienced clinical pathologist can often detect signs of in vitro aging (ie, clear, punctate cytoplasmic vacuoles vs frothy vacuolization of toxic change). Despite this, the accuracy of the provided results is unquestionably

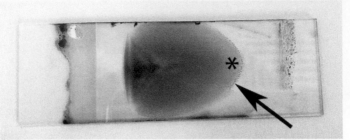

Fig. 2. Gross view of a well-made blood smear after staining. The smear has a completely stained feathered edge (*arrow*), behind which is the monolayer (*asterisk*). A feathered edge is essential for the evaluation of potential platelet clumps, larger/abnormal circulating cells, parasites, etc. Evaluation of WBC and RBC density and morphology, the WBC differential cell count, and estimation of platelets are performed in the monolayer, where cells are adequately spread and easier to identify.

affected, particularly in cases where there is a suspected inflammatory leukogram. With aged samples, some laboratories may choose to provide a comment reflecting the inaccuracy and simply enumerate all neutrophils as segmented cells and not attempt to differentiate true band neutrophils given the inherent inaccuracies in doing so. This affects a clinician's ability to know the initial severity of the inflammation and to monitor its improvement over time. Sample aging also adversely affects automated leukocyte differential counts, such as the misclassification of granulocytes as mononuclear cells.[4]

Prolonged in vitro sample aging also leads to cell rupture and pyknosis, further hindering accurate leukocyte count and differentials. This can be partially prevented by sample refrigeration. Clinical pathologists may semiquantitatively describe cell lysis by indicating the presence of few, moderate, or many "smudged" cells (**Fig. 3**) seen on blood smear evaluation. In the author's experience, neutrophils tend to lyse more readily, which can result in an artifactually decreased proportion of neutrophils and increased proportion of lymphocytes in analyzed stored samples. Lymphocytes can also swell and become vacuolated, mimicking monocytes. Pyknotic cells can be misidentified as nucleated RBCs by inexperienced personnel. Long shipping times and sample processing delays (ie, a week or more) often result in nearly all WBCs being ruptured or pyknotic, rendering the sample useless for analysis.

Red Blood Cells

As early as 12 hours after collection, RBCs take on water and swell, resulting in a falsely increased mean corpuscular volume (MCV) and decreased mean cell hemoglobin concentration (MCHC).[3,4] Although this may seem inconsequential, it has a trickle-down effect of causing a false increase in hematocrit (Hct), given that the Hct is a calculated value [a] based on the MCV and RBC count. Clinically, this can mask an anemia or hinder monitoring of an anemia. Measurement of a spun packed cell volume (PCV) does not help, because the cells are still larger and will not compact down, resulting in a falsely increased PCV. In this case, the most reliable indicator of oxygen-carrying capacity is the hemoglobin (Hgb). The Hct can be roughly estimated by multiplying the Hgb by 3.

---

[a] Hct = (RBC x MCV) ÷ 10.

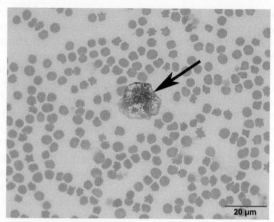

Fig. 3. Example of a "smudge cell" (*arrow*), which is a ruptured leukocyte that cannot be identified. These are seen with increased frequency in stored blood and affect accuracy of the differential count (Wright stain).

With prolonged sample storage and continued cell swelling, RBCs begin to lyse (in vitro hemolysis), resulting in a falsely decreased RBC count and Hct. This will falsely increase the MCH and MCHC, given they are denominators for Hgb in the calculations.[b] Again, Hgb should not be affected and can be used to estimate a Hct. In vitro hemolysis can occur for several other reasons, including freezing (ie, shipping in winter), difficult venipuncture, cell shearing if forcing blood through a small gauge needle (eg, when transferring into a tube), or lipemia. Lipemia due to increased very low density lipoprotein is not seen postprandially in horses and is usually due to stress or disease, most commonly in obese ponies, miniature horses, and miniature donkeys. Severe lipemia can spuriously increase the Hgb, MCH, MCHC, and total protein by refractometry.[3]

With sample aging, RBCs become depleted of adenosine triphosphate and crenated (see **Fig. 1**), possibly obscuring more significant morphologic abnormalities.

It is important to fill the EDTA tube to the "fill line," to ensure a proper ratio of EDTA to blood. If a tube is underfilled, which is typically not an issue for large animal patients, the excess EDTA will result in an osmotic draw of water from RBCs resulting in RBC shrinking and consequently a falsely decreased MCV and Hct and falsely increased MCHC. Use of a vacutainer helps prevent this error, as the appropriate volume of blood will fill based on the vacuum within the tube.[3]

Platelets

Platelet clumping is very common in horses and results in a falsely decreased count and increased mean platelet volume (MPV).[3] Platelet clumping can occur with difficult venipuncture, resulting in platelet activation, although this is typically not an issue in equine patients. Platelet clumping is frequently a result of prolonged sample storage, another reason to provide a blood smear prepared at the time of sample collection and to promptly ship samples to the diagnostic laboratory. If platelets are activated with storage, clumps would be absent on the freshly made blood smear and a reasonable platelet estimate could be provided from this smear. Although some hematology analyzers provide

[b] MCH = Hgb ÷ RBC; MCHC = (Hgb ÷ Hct) x 100.

a "flag" when platelet clumping is detected,[5] counts should always be manually verified from a blood smear. In these cases, the automated platelet count is considered a minimum but is often inaccurate and not provided with the results. Unfortunately, there are no equations to "correct" platelet counts when clumping is present.

Despite EDTA being the anticoagulant of choice for CBCs, there are reports of EDTA-dependent pseudothrombocytopenia in horses.[6,7] Approximately 5% of thrombocytopenic horses were EDTA induced in one retrospective study.[7] This phenomenon should be suspected in cases where horses have no clinical evidence of bleeding despite platelet counts being in the range where spontaneous bleeding is expected (<10,000–30,000/µL). It is important to recognize the potential for this phenomenon and avoid additional unnecessary diagnostic tests (eg, bone marrow aspiration) and immunosuppressive treatment. EDTA-dependent thrombocytopenia can be confirmed by (1) evaluating blood smears for platelet clumping and (2) comparing platelet counts in samples drawn into EDTA and heparin and/or citrate tubes at the same time point.[5–7]

Falsely increased platelet counts can also occur as a consequence of preanalytical error, some of which are avoidable. Lysed (ghost) RBCs will falsely increase platelet counts (also known as pseudothrombocytosis[4]) and yield very high MPVs. Erythrocyte lysis can occur as a result of in vitro hemolysis, as mentioned earlier, and with hemolytic anemias that have an intravascular component, for example, red maple leaf toxicity. Similarly, lipemia can falsely increase platelet counts, due to the high refractive index of lipids that is erroneously counted as platelets.[3,5]

CHEMISTRY

Biochemical testing can be performed on serum or *heparinized* plasma (green top tube). Although many biochemical panels in horses, particularly STAT testing, are performed on heparinized plasma due to the prolonged time needed for equine samples to clot (ie, about an hour), reference intervals are typically based on serum, although this may vary by laboratory. The results between these 2 sample types are mostly comparable, with the main exception being total protein and globulins, which are both higher in plasma due to the presence of fibrinogen. This difference will be more appreciable in states of inflammation, when acute phase protein concentrations are likely to be increased. Potassium results will be slightly higher in serum than plasma due to the release of potassium from platelets during clotting. This difference is mostly negligible, except in cases of marked thrombocytosis.[8] For optimal serial monitoring of a patient's results, the same sample type should be used for all analyses.

EDTA is not an appropriate anticoagulant for biochemical analysis, as it adversely affects the results of multiple different analytes. This occurs whether the sample was deliberately collected into EDTA or with inadvertent contamination of a serum or heparinized sample with EDTA. EDTA works as an anticoagulant by chelating calcium but will also chelate the other divalent cations. Thus, the main affected tests are divalent cations, such as calcium, magnesium, and iron, or enzymes that require calcium for their activity, for example, alkaline phosphatase. EDTA contamination will markedly decrease calcium and magnesium concentrations, which are often so low that they are considered "incompatible with life." If provided on the biochemical panel (iron panels are not provided by all diagnostic laboratories), iron concentrations are also markedly decreased and total iron binding capacity, a surrogate measure of transferrin (the iron transport protein), is markedly increased. Most tubes contain K_2EDTA or K_3EDTA, so these samples will also have spuriously high potassium (often > 10 mEq/L). Note that some purple top tubes contain Na_2EDTA, which will spuriously increase sodium concentrations. Spurious changes in potassium or sodium will also increase the calculated anion gap.[c]

Probably the most common preanalytical error for biochemical testing encountered in clinical pathology laboratories is submission of unseparated whole blood or delayed separation of serum or plasma from cells. This results in falsely decreased blood glucose due to the consumption and utilization of glucose by cells for metabolism.[8,9] Given the incorporation of glucose in metabolic profiles, it is important to collect and process samples properly to obtain accurate results. In addition, in horses delayed separation results in leakage of potassium from RBCs, resulting in falsely increased potassium.[8,10] Prolonged storage of whole blood also leads to spuriously high AST, LDH, CK, Mg, and phosphate.[11]

Chemistry Sample Submission to Laboratory

Blood samples for biochemical testing should be centrifuged as soon as possible after collection to harvest serum or plasma from cells. However, some time is usually required to allow clotting of equine blood in nonanticoagulant (red top) tubes, and it can be difficult to obtain serum off the clot if inadequate time is given for clotting. "Rimming the tube" or using a wooden applicator stick to separate the clot from wall of the tube can help with serum harvesting. Whole blood can be kept at room temperature for 1 hour to allow for clotting. However, it should not be left at this temperature for longer than this time, due to significant reductions in glucose concentrations.[9] For longer storage, whole blood should be kept at 4℃ and can be maintained at the temperature for up to 8 hours without significant decreases in blood glucose.[9] To harvest serum or plasma, whole blood should be centrifuged (recommended 2000 g for 10 minutes) and serum or plasma removed from cells and transferred into a separate plain tube, which should be labeled with the specimen type (and anticoagulant, if plasma). Many veterinarians use serum separator tubes that contain a gel or clot activator (ie, Corvac or tiger top tubes) to assist with harvesting serum from the clot. However, they do not prevent glucose consumption by cells, and serum must still be separated. Once separated, the sample should be shipped overnight to the diagnostic laboratory on an ice pack to ideally allow for next day testing. This is important for certain analytes, such as the hepatocellular leakage enzyme sorbitol dehydrogenase, which is only stable for 24 hours if refrigerated before significant enzyme activity decreases.[12] Otherwise, most analytes are stable in serum or heperanized plasma for 3 days when kept refrigerated.[13] If a longer delay in testing is anticipated, samples should be frozen in a dedicated (not frost-free) freezer.

CYTOLOGY

Cytologic samples include fine-needle aspirates, swabs, skin scrapes, impression smears, and body fluids. The method of sample collection (eg, endotracheal tube or transtracheal wash) and a succinct clinical history, including a description of the sampled site, as appropriate, should be provided on the request form. Provision of the latter helps the clinical pathologist interpret the cytologic findings in the context of the clinical picture and yields the most useful results. Although cytology can occasionally provide a definitive diagnosis, in most cases it narrows down the list of differential diagnoses and helps to direct further diagnostic testing (eg, culture, histopathology). Nondiagnostic results can occur with low cellularity samples and mishandled or poorly prepared samples.

---

[c] Anion gap = $(Na + K) - (HCO_3 + Cl)$.

General Principles

Regardless of the method of sample collection, there are several general principles to follow when submitting samples for cytologic evaluation. In regard to staining, Diff-Quik staining can be performed in the clinic to ensure a diagnostic sample was obtained (ie, not acellular or blood only) or to determine if additional aspirates are needed. However, it is recommended to stain the least cellular/lowest quality smear, leaving the remaining slides to be stained by the laboratory. Although Diff-Quik stains can be of high quality, staining quality is highly variable (**Figs. 4** and **5**) and more dependent on user technique, as compared with automated strainers used in diagnostic laboratories. It is important to follow the test directions for optimal staining, but for thick specimens, longer staining time is needed. Diff-Quik–stained smears are suboptimal for evaluation of mast cells and granular lymphocytes, because granules do not stain well. In addition, Diff-Quik makes it difficult to differentiate between immature and mature lymphocytes due to uniform chromatin features and is not recommended for samples from lymphoid tissues. Note that cytologic smears should be rapidly air-dried (hairdryer method given earlier) but do not need heat fixing before staining.

After preparation of the cytologic smear, regardless of the sample type, it is important to label the slide in pencil with the patient's name and sampled site. This prevents the potential preanalytical error of mixing up slides with patients at the clinic and allows for an additional quality check at the laboratory, where the slide is matched to the submitted request form. Labeling slides are particularly important when multiple sites are sampled, to ensure that the relevant cytologic reports correspond to the correct site.

In preparation for shipping, glass slides should be placed in a protective container (ie, plastic or cardboard slide holder) to prevent breaking during transit. It is also important to prevent exposure of the prepared cytologic slides from formalin fumes, if shipping with samples for histopathology. Formalin fumes alter staining properties resulting in the entire sample appearing as a fairly uniform blue/green color (**Fig. 6**) hindering evaluation of exfoliated cells. It is best practice to ship cytologic and histopathologic samples separately, because even tightly sealed containers can leak formalin fumes and damage nearby cytologic samples.

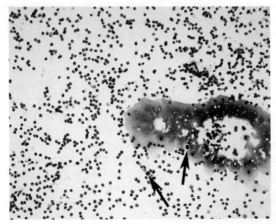

Fig. 4. Example of an overstained Diff-Quik smear. In this poorly cellular aspirate, it is difficult to see the contrast between nucleated cells (*arrows*) and the background blood at low power (20x) examination.

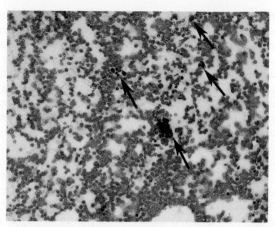

Fig. 5. Example of a well-stained Diff-Quik smear from the same aspirate as in **Fig. 4**. With the appropriate tinctorial properties, nucleated cells (*arrows*) are much easier to spot at low power (20x) in the poorly cellular smear.

Fine-Needle Aspiration

Fine-needle aspiration (FNA) with cytologic evaluation is a minimally invasive means of investigating masses, effusions, or abnormal organs. Either the aspiration (syringe attached to apply negative pressure) or nonaspiration/stab (needle only) techniques can be used.[14] The aspiration technique is ideal for masses that are firm on palpation or for suspected fluid-filled masses. The negative pressure used to exfoliate cells should be released before the needle exits the lesion to avoid aspirating material into the barrel of the syringe, where it cannot be retrieved. After aspiration, the syringe is removed from the needle. The nonaspiration or stab technique is ideal for lymph nodes, in which cells are fragile and commonly rupture with excessive negative syringe pressure, and for small, raised cutaneous masses. With either method, the needle is reattached to a syringe with several mL of air, to provide the force needed to

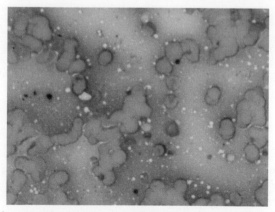

Fig. 6. Example of a stained cytologic smear that has been exposed to formalin fumes, as evident by the uniform blue to green appearance of the cells. This hinders morphologic evaluation of cells as their normal tinctorial properties are lost (Wright stain, 100x magnification).

expel the contents of the aspirate, often in the hub of the needle onto a slide. Ideally the sample should be placed onto more than one slide and gently spread (see below). If the lesion is cystic or fluid is aspirated, the fluid should be placed into EDTA for cytology and a red top tube for possible culture. (See *Fluid analysis* section later for more details). Fluid from such lesions is often of low cellularity and rarely diagnostic, as it usually contains only low numbers of macrophages. Thus, it is prudent to also aspirate more solid portions of the lesion if possible, to obtain a higher cell yield. If the aspirate and needle is bloody, it is best to dab the blood off the needle onto multiple slides first, before expelling the aspirate contents onto fresh slides. This prevents an overly hemodilute and thick smear, which also can hinder evaluation of cellular morphologic details. The bloody smears can also be smeared and submitted along with the aspirate contents. Multiple aspirates may be performed from a single lesion, and it is recommended to submit more than one smear to optimize the possibility of a diagnostic sample. Typically, 3 to 5 smears are sufficient, with more than 5 smears being excessive. Keep in mind some laboratories charge extra for examining more smears.

Aspirated contents should be expelled just in front of the frosted edge of the smear, which is approximately one-fourth of the way along the slide. Afterward, it is crucial to use another slide to gently, without added pressure, spread the aspirated material to form a monolayer in what is called a "squash" smear (**Fig. 7**). The squash preparation is the recommended method to spread FNA samples. To do this, the spreader slide is usually oriented parallel to the sample slide. The spreader slide is then placed directly on top of the sample slide and then smoothly pulled away while maintaining even contact, but not pressure, with the sample slide throughout. The sample slide is not moved in the opposite direction during this procedure to decrease force on the cells. Just expelling contents onto a slide without spreading results in a "splat smear" (**Fig. 8**), in which the droplets are often too thick to examine, precluding adequate cytologic evaluation of the morphologic features of the aspirated cells. Cells within the droplets will not spread well, appearing smaller or cannot be identified, which can skew a cytologic interpretation. On the other extreme, when excessive pressure

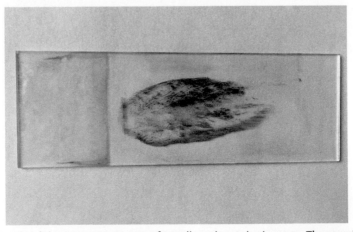

Fig. 7. Example of the gross appearance of a well-made cytologic smear. The sample was obtained via fine-needle aspirate. A spreader slide was used to spread the expelled contents, resulting in their coalescing into an oval shape with a monolayer of cells. This is known as a "squash" smear.

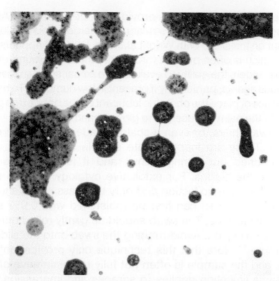

Fig. 8. Example of a "splat" smear, in which there are multiple thick droplets of material. This is the result of not using a slide to spread the expelled contents of a fine-needle aspirate. The droplets of material are too thick, which hinders morphologic evaluation of cells (Wright stain, 4x magnification).

is applied with the spreader slide, this results in cell rupture and nuclear streaming (**Fig. 9**), which results in a nondiagnostic sample.

Swabs

Smears prepared from swabbed tissue (ie, exfoliative cytology) should only be used when other collection methods are not feasible, such as for ears and ulcerated skin lesions. They are often used for endometrial cytology, although swabs yielded the lowest quality sample in one study due to marked rupturing of cells.[15] In the latter study, samples

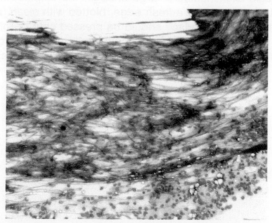

Fig. 9. Example of a cytologic smear with abundant ruptured cells and nuclear streaming. This is a consequence of excessive pressure being applied to the spreader slide during the preparation of a squash smear (Wright stain, 10x magnification).

obtained with a uterine brush consistently provided the best sample.[15] Another common impediment to diagnostic uterine swab smears is the large amount of lubricant material that is often present on the slide. With Wright staining, lubricant appears as dark purple, granular material, which is often present throughout the background of the smear and overlying cells. This hinders the ability to evaluate the smear and can mask inflammatory cells and/or infectious agents, particularly if present in low numbers. To minimize this, use a guarded swab device or place the obstetric lubricant on the back of the gloved hand and guard the swab with the palm surface of the gloved hand.

Occasionally a swab, hairs, or even a scalpel blade placed in an empty tube are directly submitted. These are inappropriate sample submissions, as any cellular material will have dried out during transit and it is hazardous for laboratory personnel to handle the blades. For exfoliative cytology, smears should be prepared at the time of sample collection and only the glass slides should be submitted. For dry lesions, the swab can first be moistened with 0.9% saline, which is unnecessary for moist lesions. The swab should be gently rolled onto a slide immediately after sample collection. Avoid rubbing the swab onto the slide, because this results in cell rupture.[14] Note that this technique only provides information as to surface changes, and the sample is often not fully representative of the underlying pathology. The same limitation applies to scrapes and impression smears of skin lesions. If a scab is present, removing it before swabbing or pressing a clean glass slide onto the lesion (ie, an impression smear) is more likely to yield a diagnostic sample. The underside of the scab can also be imprinted.[16] For the work-up of most dermatologic diseases, surgical biopsy with histopathologic examination is preferred over cytologic sampling techniques, as it provides the most information regarding lesion morphology and tissue architecture.

Impression Smears

In addition to flat skin lesions, impression smears of surgical biopsy samples with cytologic evaluation can allow for a preliminary diagnosis while histopathologic results are pending. A clean pair of forceps should be used to handle the biopsied tissue to prevent potential contamination with microorganisms or tissue from another patient. It is also important to handle the tissue carefully to prevent crush artifact, which will affect histopathologic examination. If large enough, the biopsied tissue should be cut with a clean scalpel to create a fresh edge, blotted with clean gauze to remove excessive blood, then the cut surface should be pressed onto or rolled over several glass slides 2 to 3 times each (**Fig. 10**).[14] A cut surface is more likely to provide a diagnostic sampling of the underlying pathology, as opposed to an impression of the mass

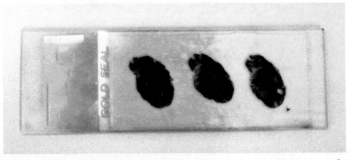

Fig. 10. Example of the gross appearance of a well-made impression smear after staining. Multiple side-by-side imprints are made from the biopsied tissue.

surface, which often just reflects surface tissue, such as inflammation with possible secondary bacterial infection.[14]

Fluid Analysis

There is a wide array of fluids that can be submitted for cytologic evaluation including body cavity fluids (ie, pleural, peritoneal, pericardial), synovial fluid, airway samples (ie, tracheal wash, bronchoalveolar lavage), cerebrospinal fluid (CSF), and fluid from aspirated masses. Regardless of the fluid type, the sample should be placed into EDTA for cytologic evaluation for optimal cellular preservation during storage. Note, that EDTA is bacteriostatic and not appropriate for culture.

A direct smear (ie, squash smear) should also be prepared at the time of sample collection and submitted along with the EDTA tube. Prolonged storage results in neutrophil nuclear swelling and the artifactual appearance of degenerative changes. Cells can also completely lyse, becoming unrecognizable. In addition, neutrophils and macrophages can quickly phagocytize RBCs and bacteria in vitro, which complicates the cytologic interpretation of hemorrhage and sepsis, respectively. Because of its inherent low cellularity, CSF does not yield useful direct smears and is generally submitted in EDTA alone. It is important to not concentrate/centrifuge fluid samples before submission to the laboratory, as this will skew automated cell counts and confound the clinical pathologist's interpretation.

General sample handling tips:

- Place blood and fluid samples into an EDTA (purple top) tube.

- Make a blood smear or direct smear of a fluid at the time of sample collection and submit it along with the EDTA tube. Rapidly air dry smears. Keep the tubes cool (refrigerate and ship on ice packs). Slides should be kept at room temperature.

- Place blood for chemistry into a nonanticoagulant (red top), serum separator, or heparin (green top) tube.

- Do not leave chemistry samples out at room temperature for more than 1 hour.

- If unable to centrifuge samples and separate serum or plasma from cells within an hour, refrigerate the sample and separate sample as soon as possible.

- Do not submit whole blood samples for chemistry testing. This includes samples in serum separator tubes. Ship separated serum or heparinized plasma in plain tubes on ice packs.

- Freeze serum or plasma if more than a 3 day delay in testing anticipated.

- Prepare a gentle squash smear of FNA samples, rather than a "splat smear." Rapidly air dry.

- Label all submitted specimens with the patient name and specimen type.

- Provide a succinct relevant clinical history and description of sampled site on the request form.

- Ship samples overnight to the diagnostic laboratory.

- Ship clinical pathologic samples and slides separately from formalin containers.

SUMMARY/DISCUSSION

You can get the most bang for your (or rather your client's) buck with clinical pathologic testing by following the sample handling recommendations provided in this article. The quality of results are directly related to the quality of the submitted samples, the onus of which is on you, the clinician, not your client.

DISCLOSURE

The author has nothing to disclose.

REFERENCES

1. Vap LM, Harr KE, Arnold JE, et al. ASVCP quality assurance guidelines: control of preanalytical and analytical factors for hematology for mammalian and nonmammalian species, hemostasis, and crossmatching in veterinary laboratories. Vet Clin Pathol 2012;41(1):8–17.
2. Gunn-Christie RG, Flatland B, Friedrichs KR, et al. ASVCP quality assurance guidelines: Control of preanalytical, analytical, and postanalytical factors for urinalysis, cytology, and clinical chemistry in veterinary laboratories. Vet Clin Pathol 2012;41(1):18–26.
3. Harvey JW. Veterinary hematology: a diagnostic guide and color atlas. St Louis (MO): Elsevier Saunders; 2012.
4. Clark P, Mogg TD, Tvedten HW, et al. Artifactual changes in equine blood following storage, detected using the advia 120 hematology analyzer. Vet Clin Pathol 2002;31(2):90–4.
5. Zandecki M, Genevieve F, Gerard J, et al. Spurious counts and spurious results on haematology analysers: a review. Part I: Platelets. Int J Lab Hematol 2007;29(1):4–20.
6. Hinchcliff KW, Kociba GJ, Mitten LA. Diagnosis of EDTA-dependent pseudothrombocytopenia in a horse. J Am Vet Med Assoc 1993;203(12):1715–6.
7. Hubers E, Bauer N, Fey K, et al. Thrombocytopenia in horses. Tierarztl Prax Ausg G Grosstiere Nutztiere 2018;46(2):73–9 [in German].
8. Stockham SL, Scott MA. Fundamentals of veterinary clinical pathology. 2nd edition. Ames (IA): Blackwell Publishing; 2008.
9. Collicutt NB, Garner B, Berghaus RD, et al. Effect of delayed serum separation and storage temperature on serum glucose concentration in horse, dog, alpaca, and sturgeon. Vet Clin Pathol 2015;44(1):120–7.
10. Muylle E, Van den Hende C, Nuytten J, et al. Potassium concentration in equine red blood cells: normal values and correlation with potassium levels in plasma. Equine Vet J 1984;16(5):447–9.
11. Rendle DI, Heller J, Hughes KJ, et al. Stability of common biochemistry analytes in equine blood stored at room temperature. Equine Vet J 2009;41(5):428–32.
12. Horney BS, Honor DJ, MacKenzie A, et al. Stability of sorbitol dehydrogenase activity in bovine and equine sera. Vet Clin Pathol 1993;22(1):5–9.
13. Thoresen SI, Havre GN, Morberg H, et al. Effects of storage time on chemistry results from canine whole blood, heparinized whole blood, serum and heparinized plasma. Vet Clin Pathol 1992;21(3):88–94.
14. Tyler RD, Cowell RL, MacAllister CG, et al. Introduction. In: Cowell RL, Tyler RD, editors. Diagnostic cytology and hematology of the horse. 2nd edition. St Louis (MO): Mosby; 2002. p. 1–9.
15. Bohn AA, Ferris RA, Mccue PM. Comparison of equine endometrial cytology samples collected with uterine swab, uterine brush, and low-volume lavage from healthy mares. Vet Clin Pathol 2014;43(4):594–600.
16. Tyler RD, Meinkoth JH, Cowell RL, et al. Cutaneous and subcutaneous lesions: masses, cysts, and fistulous tracts. In: Cowell RL, Tyler RD, editors. Diagnostic cytology and hematology of the horse. 2nd edition. St Louis (MO): Mosby; 2002. p. 19–22.

Hematology Red Flags
The Value of Blood Smear Examination in Horses

Tracy Stokol, BVSc, PhD

KEYWORDS

- Equine • Hemogram • Leukocytes • Anemia • Inflammation • Pancytopenia
- Leukemia • Lymphoma

KEY POINTS

- Hematologic numerical results provide red flags as to the presence of underlying disease.
- Examination of a blood smear for morphologic changes, for example, left shift, toxic change, abnormal cells, or infectious agents, is a crucial part of a diagnostic workup; do not rely only on numbers alone.
- Interpret laboratory data with pertinent clinical information (history, physical examination, and diagnostic imaging).

Blood is our window into the animal. From clinical pathologic results, we can identify pathologic abnormalities, involved organ(s), or the primary disease. Examination of a fresh, well-made blood smear, with recognition of clues of underlying pathology, is an important part of equine practice. Do not just look at numbers (albeit helpful); always look at a smear, because numbers do not give all the answers. Changes in morphologic features can be critical for disease diagnosis. This article uses specific case examples of hematologic numerical and morphologic changes that are red flags or clues to underlying disease.

CASE 1

A 21-year-old Quarter Horse mare presented with fever, inappetence, and limb edema. The mare was tachycardic, tachypneic, and febrile, with injected sclera, hyperemic, and tacky mucous membranes, prolonged capillary refill time, and skin tenting. Pertinent results are shown.

Department of Population Medicine and Diagnostic Sciences, Cornell University, College of Veterinary Medicine, S1-058 Schurman Hall, Upper Tower Road, Ithaca, NY 14853-6401, USA
E-mail address: tracy.stokol@cornell.edu

Vet Clin Equine 36 (2020) 15–33
https://doi.org/10.1016/j.cveq.2019.11.001
0749-0739/20/© 2019 Elsevier Inc. All rights reserved.

Case 1: Hemogram				
Test Name	Result		Reference Interval	Units
Hematocrit (HCT)	86	(H)	34–46	%
Red blood cells (RBC)	15.8	(H)	6.6–9.7	× 10⁶/µL
Mean cell volume (MCV)	54		43–55	fL
Mean cell hemoglobin concentration (MCHC)	34		34–37	g/dL
White blood cells (WBC)	1.4	(L)	5.2–10.1	× 10³/µL
Segmented neutrophils	0.5	(L)	2.7–6.6	× 10³/µL
Band neutrophils	0.2	(H)	0–0.1	× 10³/µL
Lymphocytes	0.4	(L)	1.2–4.9	× 10³/µL
Platelets	57	(L)	94–232	× 10³/µL
Mean platelet volume	7.5		5.3–8.4	fL
Fibrinogen (heat precipitation)	400	(H)	0–200	g/dL
WBC examination	See **Fig. 1.**			

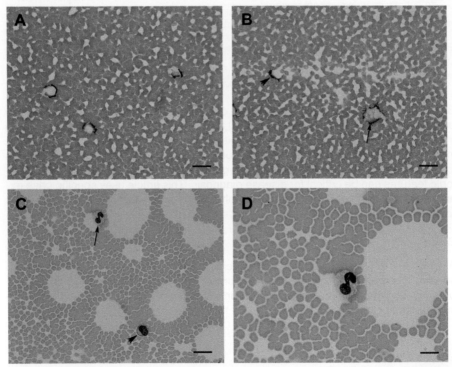

Fig. 1. Case 1, a 21-year-old Quarter Horse mare with erythrocytosis, leukopenia, and thrombocytopenia (modified Wright's stain). It can be difficult to find a good area to examine neutrophil morphology in these horses. (*A*) Neutrophils often blow out and are hard to identify. (*B*) A monocyte (*arrow*) and lymphocyte (*arrowhead*). (*C*) Where morphology is better preserved, a band neutrophil (*arrow*) and lymphocyte (*arrowhead*) can be identified (bar = 20 µm, A–C). (*D*) The band neutrophil is moderately toxic (Döhle bodies, cytoplasmic basophilia) (bar = 10 µm).

Case 1: Plasma Biochemistry				
Test Name	Result		Reference Interval	Units
Sodium	137		134–142	mEq/L
Potassium	3.0		2.4–4.8	mEq/L
Chloride	84	(L)	95–104	mEq/L
Bicarbonate	15	(L)	24–31	mEq/L
Anion gap	41	(H)	12–19	mEq/L
Urea nitrogen	30	(H)	10–22	mg/dL
Creatinine	3.5	(H)	0.8–1.5	mg/dL
Albumin	2.5	(L)	2.9–3.6	g/dL
Glucose	196	(H)	71–122	mg/dL

Case 1 Red Flags

1. Marked erythrocytosis: A HCT of 86% is a marked erythrocytosis and a red flag. There are several causes of erythrocytosis (**Fig. 2**), but a marked increase

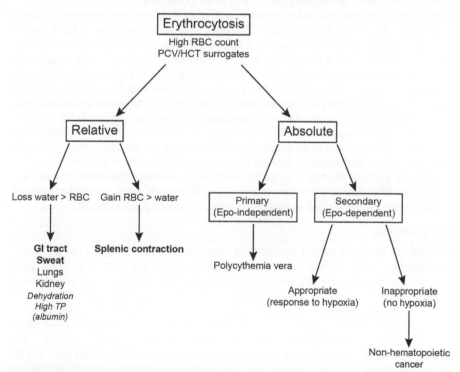

Fig. 2. Mechanisms of erythrocytosis. Erythrocytosis (increased RBCs, with packed cell volume (PCV)/HCT used as RBC surrogates) can be relative, from extracellular fluid loss (hemoconcentration) or splenic contraction.[29,36] Fluid loss from the gastrointestinal (GI) tract (eg, sequestration, diarrhea) or sweating is most common and is identified by dehydration or increased total protein (TP), specifically albumin, concentrations. An absolute erythrocytosis can be erythropoietin (Epo)-independent or -dependent. Primary erythrocytosis is usually a chronic leukemia, polycythemia vera, but may be congenital.[52] Secondary erythrocytosis can be appropriate with hypoxia (eg, respiratory disease[53]) or inappropriate with high erythropoietin or epinephrine owing to tumors.[6,7,54]

(>65%) is usually due to gastrointestinal (GI) disease, specifically conditions causing copious fluid sequestration in the upper GI tract (eg, gastric rupture,[1] proximal duodenitis–jejunitis,[2] ileus[3]) or colon (eg, colonic torsion[4]), or fluid losses with diarrhea (eg, *Neorickettsia risticii*[5]). It is associated with a poor prognosis.[2,5] An absolute erythrocytosis is a rare, typically paraneoplastic, condition,[6,7] and should be suspected when a high HCT is not alleviated by appropriate fluid therapy. Note that a mild fluid-unresponsive erythrocytosis (48%–56%) has been observed anecdotally in horses with severe liver disease or failure.

2. Severe leukopenia owing to a neutropenia with a left shift and toxic change: This leukogram is characteristic of severe acute inflammation, which is usually due to inflammatory or necrotizing GI disorders, with absorption of bacterial toxins.[1,2] Although neutropenia with a left shift on a hemogram suggests inflammation, identification of toxic change is crucial for confirmation, because mild neutropenia can occur with sample storage, presumably from cell lysis in vitro. There are other leukogram patterns of inflammation (**Fig. 3**) and some horses with mild or established inflammation may have normal hemogram results. Measurement of serum amyloid A, a sensitive major acute phase protein,[8,9] would be useful in such horses. However, increases in serum amyloid A concentrations may not be seen with localized (eg, inflammatory airway disease[10]) or chronic conditions.

3. Moderate thrombocytopenia: Thrombocytopenia is uncommon, with an incidence of 1% to 3% (<75 or 90 × 10³/µL).[11,12] There are several mechanisms for thrombocytopenia (**Fig. 4**), but it is usually due to inflammation (usually in the GI tract) or infectious agents, such *Anaplasma phagocytophilum*.[13,14] Horses with *Anaplasma* frequently do not have a left shift or toxic change, but may be neutropenic and/or mildly anemic.[13] Morulae can be seen in neutrophils (**Fig. 5**), but are not always present, and targeted polymerase chain reaction testing on whole blood is recommended in suspect cases. A moderate to severe thrombocytopenia (<50 × 10³/µL) is unusual for *Anaplasma* and, in the absence of inflammation or positive *Anaplasma* results, would raise suspicion for underlying neoplasia.[15,16] An antibody-mediated pseudothrombocytopenia can occur in EDTA-anticoagulated blood,[11,17] however, platelet clumps are usually identified in smears, illustrating the need to verify platelet counts by smear examination. If this artifact is suspected, platelet counts can be rechecked in citrate- or heparin-anticoagulated blood.

Case 1 Summary

Hematologic changes reflect severe fluid sequestration, leading to marked hemoconcentration, and severe inflammation (neutropenia, left shift, moderate toxic change, hyperfibrinogenemia, and hypoalbuminemia) with likely concurrent nonovert disseminated intravascular coagulation (thrombocytopenia). The most helpful result on the biochemical panel is metabolic alkalosis (disproportionately low chloride vs sodium), which indicates chloride sequestration in the upper GI tract. These blood results, with no gastric reflux, should raise suspicion for a gastric rupture.[1] The biochemical panel also revealed a primary titration acidosis (high anion gap, low bicarbonate), likely L-lactic acidosis, with the acidosis dominating. There is prerenal and possibly renal azotemia, stress (hyperglycemia, lymphopenia), and GI albumin losses.

An idiopathic gastric rupture was found after humane euthanasia. Gastric rupture can be secondary to any condition causing severe fluid accumulation and distension of the upper GI tract (eg, ileus, strangulating obstruction, anterior enteritis). In a retrospective report of 47 cases, 24 were idiopathic, 20 were from impaction, and 3 had perforated ulcers. Affected horses had higher heart and respiratory rates, packed

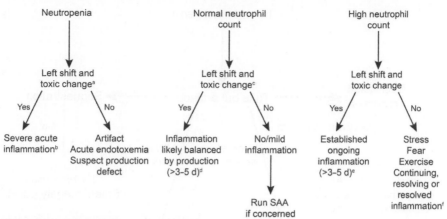

Fig. 3. Neutrophil leukogram patterns. Neutropenia (usually severe) with a left shift (often degenerative, ie, more immature than mature neutrophils) and toxic change is characteristic of a severe acute inflammatory leukogram. Mild neutropenia can be a storage-associated artifact. Moderate to severe neutropenia without a left shift could be from acute endotoxemia[55] or a production defect (particularly with other cytopenias). There may be a left shift and toxic change if there is concurrent inflammation. A normal neutrophil count with a left shift and toxic change implies the marrow is responding to existing inflammation. A single hemogram is a snapshot in time and serial testing is recommended to determine if the inflammation is resolving or worsening. A normal neutrophil count with no left shift or toxic change does not rule out underlying inflammation and measurement of serum amyloid A (SAA) can be done if clinically indicated. Neutrophilia with a mild left shift and no to mild toxic change indicates established ongoing inflammation and may be accompanied by a monocytosis. Neutrophilia alone usually indicates mild inflammation, resolving inflammation or rebound after resolved inflammation or acute endotoxemia. However, mild neutrophilia (<12 × 10³/μL) can be due to corticosteroids,[56,57] exercise,[29] or extreme excitement/fear.[30] [a] Left shift may be degenerative (immature > mature) or nondegenerative (mature > immature neutrophils). Toxic change is usually moderate to severe with a degenerative left shift. Monitoring of leukogram changes every 24 hours is recommended to document resolution. [b] Concurrent production defect cannot be ruled out, but is uncommon. [c] Left shift is usually not degenerative. If degenerative, it indicates inflammation is overwhelming production. [d] The normal neutrophil count suggests that the bone marrow has had time to mount a response to the inflammation (granulocytic hyperplasia); however, this response may be insufficient. Monitoring of leukogram changes every 24 hours is recommended to determine ifinflammation is resolving or worsening. There may be a concurrent monocytosis (disease dependent). [e] The bone marrow has responded and is combating the inflammation, but inflammation is still present. The left shift is usually mild (if present and is often called a regenerative left shift), as is toxic change. It may be accompanied by a monocytosis, depending on the cause of inflammation. Can monitor with sensitive, rapidly changing acute phase markers, such as SAA. [f] The degree of neutrophilia can guide as to continuing inflammation or stress. Stress (endogenous glucocorticoids), exercise or fear (the latter two are likely epinephrine-mediated) rarely increases neutrophils >12 × 10³/μL in horses. Measurement of SAA can help to distinguish between stress and inflammation, unless the inflammation has resolved. Extreme exercise can induce a transient neutrophilia (and lymphocytosis).

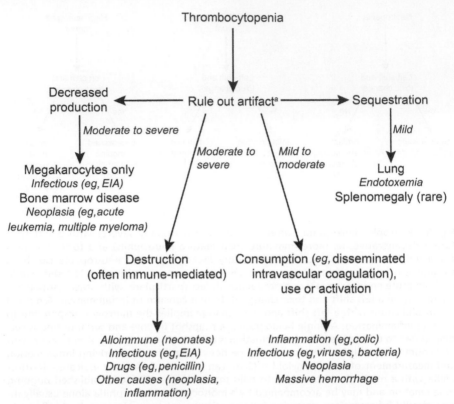

Fig. 4. Mechanisms of thrombocytopenia. The degree of thrombocytopenia (mild, 50–95 × 10³/μL; moderate, 30–50 × 10³/μL; severe, <30 × 10³/μL) provides clues as to the mechanism, although multiple mechanisms may be operative in a given patient. Counts should be verified by smear examination; clumping decreases the count. Clumping is usually from collection- or storage-associated activation, however, a naturally occurring antibody can bind platelets in EDTA, inducing clumping. [a] Owing to platelet clumping. Always examine a blood smear for clumps to verify any platelet count. EIA, equine infectious anemia.

cell volume and lactate concentrations, and lower leukocyte counts, than generic colic controls. More affected horses had systemic inflammatory response syndrome and none survived.[1]

Key Points

- Marked erythrocytosis (HCT/packed cell volume of >65%) is usually due to GI fluid losses or sequestration and is a poor prognostic indicator.
- Marked neutropenia with a left shift, often degenerative, and moderate to marked toxic change is classic for a severe acute inflammatory leukogram. Look for the source of inflammation (often GI).
- Neutropenia without a left shift or toxic change can be a storage artifact.
- Verify platelet counts by smear examination (clumps will lower counts).
- Thrombocytopenia is usually due to inflammation or infection. Rare causes include pseudothrombocytopenia, immune-mediated thrombocytopenia, and cancer.

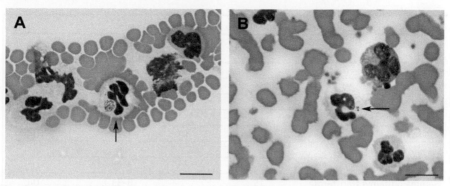

Fig. 5. *Anaplasma phagocytophilum* morulae. (*A*) Morulae (*arrow*) can be found within neutrophils, particularly at the feathered edge. (*B*) With treatment or prolonged storage, morulae can degrade and condense (*arrow*), becoming difficult to identify (modified Wright's stain; bar = 10 μm).

- In relevant geographic areas, look for *Anaplasma* morulae in smears and consider polymerase chain reaction or serologic testing in horses with compatible symptoms (eg, fever, stiff gait, and limb and subcutaneous edema).[13,14]

CASE 2

A 12-year-old Quarter Horse gelding presented with a 3- to 4-day history of colic, fever, and anorexia. The horse had been given penicillin 3 weeks earlier for a leg laceration, which was switched to trimethoprim-sulfonamides. The gelding was quiet, tachycardic, and febrile, with icteric mucosa and the urine was dark red. Pertinent results are shown.

Test Name	Result		Reference Interval	Units
Case 2: Hemogram				
HCT	17	(L)	34–46	%
RBC	6.5	(L)	6.6–9.7	× 10⁶/μL
MCV	53		43–55	fL
MCHC	37		34–37	g/dL
Red cell distribution width (RDW)	21.7	(H)	16.3–19.3	%
WBC	18.3	(H)	5.2–10.1	× 10³/μL
Segmented neutrophils	17.4	(H)	2.7–6.6	× 10³/μL
Band neutrophils	0.0		0	× 10³/μL
Lymphocytes	0.6	(L)	1.2–4.9	× 10³/μL
Platelets	413	(H)	94–232	× 10³/μL
Mean platelet volume	7.9		5.3–8.4	fL
RBC examination	See **Fig. 6**.			
Plasma appearance	Moderate icterus, slight hemolysis			

Case 2: Plasma Biochemistry				
Test Name	Result		Reference Interval	Units
Total protein	8.2	(H)	5.4–7.0	g/dL
Albumin	2.8	(L)	2.9–3.6	g/dL
Globulins	5.4	(H)	2.3–3.8	g/dL
Creatinine	1.6		0.9–1.8	mg/dL
Aspartate aminotransferase	678	(H)	222–489	U/L
Sorbitol dehydrogenase	6		1–6	U/L
Glutamate dehydrogenase	7		2–10	U/L
Gamma glutamyl transferase	15		8–33	U/L
Total bilirubin	7.1	(H)	0.5–2.1	mg/dL
Direct bilirubin	0.2		0.1–0.3	mg/dL
Indirect bilirubin	6.9	(H)	0.3–2.0	mg/dL
Creatine kinase	2468	(H)	171–567	U/L
Lipemia	17		<20	Units
Hemolysis	43		<20	Units
Icterus	10			Units

Voided urinalysis: 1.013 specific gravity, 8 pH, 100 mg/dL (2+) proteinuria, and 4+ blood. The sediment lacked cells or casts.

Case 2 Red Flags

1. Severe anemia (<20% HCT/packed cell volume): This is uncommon in adult horses, but can be due to hemorrhage, hemolysis (reduced in vivo RBC life-span), or decreased production. History, physical examination findings, smear evaluation for RBC morphologic changes, and other clinical pathologic results can help to distinguish between mechanisms (**Fig. 7**). In my experience, acute

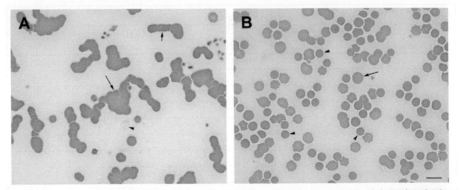

Fig. 6. Case 2, a 12-year-old Quarter Horse gelding with severe anemia. (*A*) In the thicker part of the smear, there are 3-dimensional RBC aggregates (agglutination, *long arrow*), and longitudinal RBC stacks (rouleaux formation, *short arrow*). A few RBC ghosts, indicating intravascular hemolysis (*arrowhead*), and platelet clumps are present. (*B*) In the monolayer, there are several macrocytes, supporting regeneration (*arrow*), and smaller darker RBCs, presumptive spherocytes (*arrowheads*) (modified Wright's stain; bar = 10 μm).

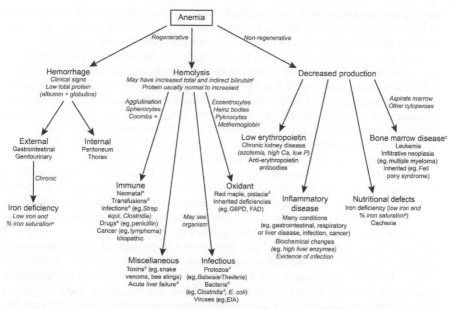

Fig. 7. Mechanisms and causes of anemia. Anemia can be due to hemorrhage, hemolysis or decreased production. The first 2 mechanisms are usually regenerative and can be distinguished by documenting hemorrhage and low total protein concentration. Chronic external blood loss can deplete iron stores, resulting in iron deficiency, but this has not been reported in horses. Hemolytic anemia is caused by premature RBC destruction via extravascular hemolysis (macrophage phagocytosis), with some disorders causing concurrent intravascular hemolysis (RBC lysis). Agglutination, spherocytes, and a positive Coombs test support an immune-mediated anemia, which can be idiopathic or secondary to blood group incompatibilities, infectious agents, drugs, or cancer.[20,28,58–62] Ingestion of wilted red maple or *Pistacia* leaves causes an oxidant-induced hemolytic anemia, with eccentrocytes, Heinz bodies, pyknocytes (RBC remnants formed from eccentrocytes), and methemoglobinemia.[27,63] Inherited RBC defects, infectious agents, acute liver failure, and envenomation (bees, snakes) can cause a hemolytic anemia. Production defects usually result in mild to moderate nonregenerative anemias and are due to inflammatory disease[2,22–24] or, less commonly, chronic kidney disease.[64] Bone marrow disease should be suspected with moderate to severe nonregenerative anemias or if there are other cytopenias (neutropenia, thrombocytopenia). Severe anemia alone is rare and due to inherited defects, for example, Fell pony syndrome, or anti-erythropoietin antibody production after treatment with human recombinant erythropoietin.[50,65] E. coli, *Escherichia coli*; EIA, equine infectious anemia; G6PD, glucose-6-phosphate dehydrogenase; FAD, flavin adenine nucleotide. [a] Inflammation can also result in these changes in iron. [b] Foals with neonatal isoerythrolysis can have increased direct (conjugated) and indirect (unconjugated) bilirubin. [c] Usually causes multiple cytopenias versus anemia alone. [d] Can have concurrent intravascular hemolysis.

intra-abdominal hemorrhage, prolonged external hemorrhage (eg, guttural pouch mycosis), and hemolysis are the more common causes of severe anemia in an adult horse in the absence of other cytopenias (neutropenia, thrombocytopenia). Hemorrhage or hemolysis induce a regenerative response within 4 to 5 days, although this depends on anemia severity (mild anemia will not stimulate a robust response) and underlying disease, which may suppress regeneration. It is difficult to confirm a regenerative response, because expected changes in a hemogram are subtle and not specific for regeneration. We look for a high MCV or RDW on numerical results and for macrocytes (larger RBCs with normal color; see **Fig. 6**B) in smears. However, macrocytes can reflect abnormal production, for example, leukemia-associated dysplasia.[18] The RDW and MCV will only be increased if there are enough macrocytes. A high RDW can be due to smaller RBCs, whereas a high MCV is a common storage artifact.[19] Polychromatophils and nucleated RBCs are seen rarely in acute severe anemia.[20] Low numbers of reticulocytes (immature RBCs containing RNA) can be detected using fluorescent-based analyzers[21]; however, I have found these counts helpful for confirming regeneration in only a few anemic horses and such counts are not performed routinely. Nucleated RBCs can be a flag for underlying hematopoietic neoplasia (eg, acute leukemia); however, single nucleated RBCs may be of no pathologic relevance in anemic or nonanemic horses. Pyknotic leukocytes may be mistaken for nucleated RBCs in smears of stored blood. Biochemical results can help to identify underlying diseases that suppress regeneration or are the cause of a nonregenerative anemia (see **Fig. 7**).

2. Moderate neutrophilia (>13 × 10³/μL): This finding, even without a left shift or toxic change, is usually due to inflammation (see **Fig. 3**). A marked neutrophilia (>25 × 10³/μL) is infrequent and typically indicates long-standing or persistent inflammation, usually in an internal or sequestered site (eg, lungs, cardiac valves, or abdominal abscesses).[22–25] A paraneoplastic leukocytosis has not been reported in horses.

3. Moderate thrombocytosis: Thrombocytosis (>400 × 10³/μL) was identified in 1% of 2346 horses in 1 study and was associated with inflammation, with 1 suspected case of essential thrombocythemia.[26] With automated analyzers, lysed RBCs or RBC fragments can be counted as platelets; always examine a smear to verify platelet counts. In case 2, there were many platelets in the smear (see **Fig. 6**A), verifying the thrombocytosis.

Case 2 Summary

The main numerical red flag was severe anemia, which seemed to be regenerative based on moderate macrocytes and a high RDW. Informative finding on a blood smear were numerous spherocytes and RBC agglutinates, indicating an immune-mediated hemolytic anemia, which was confirmed by a positive direct Coombs test. Mild hemoglobinemia with ghost (lysed) RBCs and hemoglobinuria indicate a concurrent intravascular component (ghost RBCs and hemolyzed plasma do not always indicate intravascular hemolysis; they can be an storage artifact). Agglutination should be differentiated from rouleaux formation with a saline dilution (1:10 blood:saline) test; 3-dimensional agglutinates remain, whereas RBC stacks dispersed. Rouleaux formation can be normal in horses, but was considered excessive in this case and was attributed to inflammation (increased immunoglobulins/ fibrinogen). The neutrophilia, thrombocytosis, and hypoalbuminemia (negative acute phase protein) also supported inflammation. High total and indirect bilirubin concentrations were due to hemolytic anemia and anorexia. High aspartate aminotransferase and creatine kinase activities indicated muscle injury. Horses with intravascular hemolysis are at risk of acute kidney injury from hemoglobin- and ischemia-mediated tubular inury.[27] The 1.013 urine specific gravity and 2+ proteinuria were concerning for tubular dysfunction, despite the horse not being azotemic. The initiating cause of the immune-mediated hemolytic anemia was likely the penicillin[20] or possibly the trimethoprim-sulfonamides.[28] The horse recovered with immunosuppressive therapy (azathioprine and dexamethasone).

Key Points

- Severe anemia is uncommon and usually secondary to acute abdominal hemorrhage, persistent external hemorrhage, or hemolysis in adult horses.
- Macrocytic RBCs support regeneration, but can be due to abnormal RBC production. They may be absent or in low numbers in a mild or acute onset hemolytic or hemorrhagic anemia. Polychromatophilic RBCs are not reliably seen in regenerative anemia.
- More than 1 nucleated RBC per 100 WBCs is rare and a flag for bone marrow injury, splenic dysfunction, or cancer.
- RBC morphologic features may reveal the cause of hemolytic anemia: infectious agents, oxidant injury (eccentrocytes, Heinz bodies), or immune mediated.
- Intravascular hemolysis is characterized by hemoglobinemia, hemoglobinuria, and RBC ghosts. Hemolyzed plasma and RBC ghosts may also be due to in vitro hemolysis.
- Mild nonregenerative anemias (HCT of >25%) are typically due to chronic inflammatory disease.

CASE 3

A 15-year-old Hanoverian gelding presented with acute ataxia. Cerebrospinal fluid analysis revealed normal counts and protein, with lymphocytes dominating in a smear. Hemogram results are shown.

Case 3: Hemogram				
Test Name	Result		Reference Interval	Units
HCT	33	(L)	34–46	%
MCV	47		43–55	fL
MCHC	35		34–37	g/dL
RDW	18.5		16.3–19.3	%
WBC	18.0	(H)	5.2–10.1	$\times 10^3/\mu L$
Segmented neutrophils	9.0	(H)	2.7–6.6	$\times 10^3/\mu L$
Band neutrophils	0.0		0	$\times 10^3/\mu L$
Lymphocytes	8.7	(H)	1.2–4.9	$\times 10^3/\mu L$
Platelets	190		94–232	$\times 10^3/\mu L$
RBC examination	No significant abnormalities			
WBC examination	See **Fig. 8**			
Plasma appearance	Slight hemolysis			

Case 3 Red Flags

Mild Lymphocytosis: Lymphocytosis is uncommon in adult horses and causes include strenuous exercise,[29–31] antigenic stimulation or chronic inflammation (from infectious agents, eg, *Trypanosoma evansi*,[32] *A phagocytophilum*[33]), and mature lymphoid neoplasms (lymphoma/chronic lymphocytic leukemia).[34,35] Strenuous exercise with training or extreme excitement/fear, induces a transient physiologic small lymphocytosis,[29,31] which reach as high as 14.3 $\times 10^3/\mu L$ in young horses.[30] A mild lymphocytosis (<10.0 $\times 10^3/\mu L$) occurs with training.[29,31]

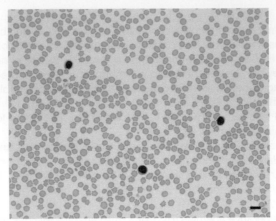

Fig. 8. Case 3, a 15-year-old Hanoverian gelding with a mild lymphocytosis. Lymphocytes were small cells, with clumped chromatin and scant blue cytoplasm (modified Wright's stain; bar = 10 μm).

Epinephrine is considered responsible; however, 2 mg epinephrine given intravenously did not alter leukocyte or differential counts in Standardbreds (the dose may not have mimicked physiologic levels).[36] Antigenic stimulation causes a mild lymphocytosis; however, the lymphocytosis with *T evansi* can be substantial ($\leq$34.0 $\times$ 10³/μL).[32] Mature B-cell neoplasms should be considered in an adult horse with a lymphocytosis,[34] particularly if no infection is identified or the lymphocytosis persists. Smear examination is important to verify that a lymphocytosis is due to mature cells and not small immature neoplastic cells or blasts, which would indicate an acute leukemia or leukemic phase of lymphoma.[18,35,37] Abnormal morphologic features, for example, irregular nuclear shapes,[34,38,39] may help to identify a neoplasm (**Fig. 9**). Foals can have higher lymphocyte counts

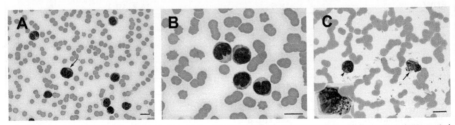

Fig. 9. Abnormal lymphocytes in horses with lymphoid neoplasia (modified Wright's stain). (*A*) Lymphocytes in a 14-year-old Clydesdale mare with a marked lymphocytosis (103.8 $\times$ 10³/μL) owing to chronic lymphocytic leukemia[34] are mostly small cells (8–10 μm) with clumped mature chromatin. Some cells have indented or lobulated nuclei. There were less than 10% large lymphocytes (*arrow*), which could be reactive or neoplastic (bar = 10 μm). (*B*) Higher magnification shows lobulated to convoluted lymphocyte nuclei (bar = 10 μm). (*C*) Despite a normal lymphocyte count, small to intermediate lymphocytes in an adult Quarter Horse gelding contained globular red cytoplasmic granules (granular lymphocyte, *arrow*; *inset*, magnified image). A few agranular small lymphocytes with deeper blue cytoplasm were presumably reactive (*arrowhead*). The dominance of granular lymphocytes were supportive of an underlying lymphoid tumor, which usually arise in the intestine or, less commonly, liver or spleen and metastasize widely.[38,66] A primary intestinal lymphoma was suspected in this horse based on low albumin concentrations (bar = 10 μm).

and more reactive-appearing lymphocytes versus adults, with counts peaking at 1 month of age (9.7 $\times$ 10^3/μL).[40,41]

Case 3 Summary

Neurologic symptoms worsened and the gelding was humanely killed. A post-mortem examination revealed generalized internal lymphadenopathy and cecal and renal masses owing to a T-cell–rich B-cell lymphoma. The lymphocytes in the cerebrospinal fluise and neurologic signs were attributed to the tumor. Viral and bacterial infections can induce a mild cerebrospinal fluid lymphocytosis[42,43]; however, these diseases usually cause lymphopenia versus lymphocytosis in blood and the latter finding was a red flag for neoplasia in this neurologic horse.

The mild nonregenerative normocytic normochromic anemia was likely due to inflammatory disease or tumor infiltrates. The mild neutrophilia could be due to inflammation, endogenous glucocorticoids, or possibly epinephrine (see **Fig. 3**).

Key Points

- Mild mature cell lymphocytosis can be due to age (<1 year old), strenuous exercise, extreme fear/excitement (young horses), antigenic stimulation from infectious agents, or lymphoid neoplasia.
- Marked mature lymphocytosis (>15 $\times$ 10^3/μL) is usually due to lymphoid neoplasia, but many affected animals will have not have a lymphocytosis.
- Examine leukocyte morphologic features to verify that lymphocytes are mature versus blasts or help support a diagnosis of lymphoid neoplasia.

CASE 4

A 2-year-old Quarter Horse gelding presented with progressive lethargy and decreased performance for 1 month. The horse was tachycardic and tachypneic with pale mucosa. Hematologic results are shown.

Case 4: Hemogram				
Test Name	Result		Reference Interval	Units
HCT	10	(L)	34–46	%
MCV	59	(H)	43–55	fL
MCHC	36		34–37	g/dL
RDW	27.6	(H)	16.3–19.3	%
WBC	4.2	(L)	5.2–10.1	$\times$ 10^3/μL
Segmented neutrophils	2.2	(L)	2.7–6.6	$\times$ 10^3/μL
Band neutrophils	0.0		0	$\times$ 10^3/μL
Lymphocytes	1.8		1.2–4.9	$\times$ 10^3/μL
Monocytes	0.1		0–0.6	$\times$ 10^3/μL
Platelets	29	(L)	94–232	$\times$ 10^3/μL
Mean plaelet volume	6.0		5.3–8.4	fL
Fibrinogen (heat precipitation)	200		0–200	g/dL
RBC examination	Moderate anisocytosis, moderate macrocytes, mild rouleaux formation			
WBC examination	See **Fig. 10**			
Plasma appearance	Normal			

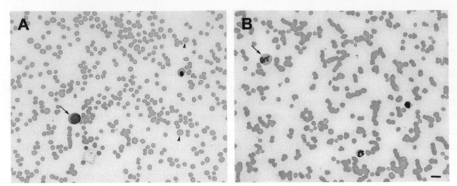

Fig. 10. Case 4, a 2-year-old Quarter Horse gelding with pancytopenia. (*A*) A few large mononuclear cells (12–15 μm) with fine chromatin (*arrow*), moderate macrocytes (*arrowheads*), and several nucleated RBCs (the other nucleated cell) were seen in the smear. (*B*) A dysplastic neutrophil (larger than normal, *arrow*) (modified Wright's stain, bar = 10 μm).

Case 4 Red Flags

Pancytopenia: A major flag, this indicates a bone marrow disorder, with rare exceptions of infectious agents (eg, *A phagocytophilum*). The most frequently reported cause of pancytopenia is neoplasia, usually acute myeloid (AML)[18] or lymphoid leukemia,[18,37,44,45] with individual reports of myelodysplastic syndrome,[46] bone marrow aplasia, or severe hypoplasia (presumed to be immune mediated),[47] multiple myeloma,[48] and myelofibrosis (cause unknown).[49] A marrow aspirate or core biopsy is indicated in pancytopenic horses with negative infectious disease testing (**Fig. 11**). Smear examination is recommended to identify blasts, a marker for underlying neoplasia. Other smear findings that may support marrow neoplasia (usually AML or myelodysplastic syndrome) are hematopoietic dysplasia (eg, giant neutrophils or platelets). However, dysplasia can be acquired (eg, drugs, nutritional deficiencies) or inherited[50,51] and is not diagnostic alone for neoplasia.

Case 4 Summary

A presumptive diagnosis of acute leukemia was made, based on blasts and dysplastic neutrophils in a smear. Macrocytosis was attributed to abnormal production and not regeneration. Serum protein electrophoresis revealed a polyclonal gammopathy. A bone marrow aspirate confirmed a leukemia, which phenotyped as AML on flow cytometric analysis.

Key Points

- Pancytopenia is usually due to underlying marrow neoplasia, particularly AML or acute lymphoid leukemia.
- Marrow aspiration or core biopsy is needed for a definitive diagnosis in pancytopenic horses.
- Examine a blood smear to look for blasts, which would support a presumptive diagnosis of marrow neoplasia.
- Blasts could be lymphoid or myeloid. Lineage identification requires additional testing, for example, immunophenotyping.
- Other clues for marrow neoplasia are hematopoietic dysplasia.
- Regardless of the cause, the prognosis in pancytopenic horses is grave.

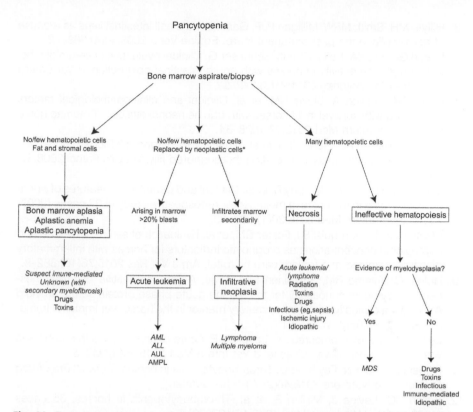

Fig. 11. Bone marrow causes of pancytopenia. Bone marrow aspirates or core biopsies in pancytopenic horses may yield the following scenarios. (1) Hypocellular or aplastic marrows consisting mostly of stromal cells (eg, fibroblasts) with few hematopoietic cells.[47] There is rare concurrent myelofibrosis[49] (always secondary, never primary). (2) Hypercellular marrows consisting of neoplastic cells (acute leukemia or an infiltrative tumor; eg, lymphoma or multiple myeloma),[18,37,44,45,48] necrosis,[45] or viable hematopoietic lineages. The latter is called ineffective hematopoiesis and if there is concurrent dysplasia, myelodysplastic syndrome, a neoplastic disorder, is favored.[46] In the absence of dysplasia, other conditions should be considered, but have not been reported to date in horses. Italicized conditions: Reported in the horse; nonitalicized conditions: Hypothetical based on other species. ALL, acute lymphoid leukemia; AMPL, acute mixed phenotype leukemia; AUL, acute undifferentiated leukemia; MDS, myelodysplasia syndrome. * Indicates extensive infiltration or effacement of normal hematopoiesis.

DISCLOSURE

The author has no conflicts of interest to disclose.

REFERENCES

1. Winfield LS, Dechant JE. Primary gastric rupture in 47 horses (1995-2011). Can Vet J 2015;56(9):953–8.

2. Seahorn TL, Cornick JL, Cohen ND. Prognostic indicators for horses with duodenitis-proximal jejunitis. 75 horses (1985-1989). J Vet Intern Med 1992; 6(6):307–11.

3. Hillyer MH, Smith MRW, Milligan PJP. Gastric and small intestinal ileus as a cause of acute colic in the post parturient mare. Equine Vet J 2008;40(4):368–72.

4. Megid Gomaa NA, Köller G, Fritz Schusser G. Clinical evaluation of serum alcohol dehydrogenase activity in horses with acute intestinal obstruction. J Vet Emerg Crit Care (San Antonio) 2011;21(3):242–52.

5. Bertin FR, Reising A, Slovis NM, et al. Clinical and clinicopathological factors associated with survival in 44 horses with equine neorickettsiosis (Potomac horse Fever). J Vet Intern Med 2013;27:1528–34.

6. Gold JR, Warren AL, French TW, et al. What is your diagnosis? Biopsy impression smear of a hepatic mass in a yearling thoroughbred filly. Vet Clin Pathol 2008;37: 339–43.

7. Luethy D, Habecker P, Murphy B, et al. Clinical and pathological features of pheo-chromocytoma in the horse: a multi-center retrospective study of 37 cases (2007-2014). J Vet Intern Med 2016;30(1):309–13.

8. Westerman TL, Tornquist SJ, Foster CM, et al. Evaluation of serum amyloid A and haptoglobin concentrations as prognostic indicators for horses with inflammatory disease examined at a tertiary care hospital. Am J Vet Res 2015;76(10):882–8.

9. Hultén C, Tulamo RM, Suominen MM, et al. A non-competitive chemilumines-cence enzyme immunoassay for the equine acute phase protein serum amyloid A (SAA) – a clinically useful inflammatory marker in the horse. Vet Immunol Immu-nopathol 1999;68(2–4):267–81.

10. Leclere M, Lavoie-Lamoureux A, Lavoie J-P. Acute phase proteins in racehorses with inflammatory airway disease. J Vet Intern Med 2015;29(3):940–5.

11. Hübers E, Bauer N, Fey K, et al. Thrombocytopenia in horses. Tierarztl Prax Ausg G Grosstiere Nutztiere 2018;46(2):73–9 [in German].

12. Sellon DC, Levine J, Millikin E, et al. Thrombocytopenia in horses: 35 cases (1989-1994). J Vet Intern Med 1996;10:127–32.

13. Madigan JE, Gribble D. Equine ehrlichiosis in Northern California: 49 cases (1968-1981). J Am Vet Med Assoc 1987;190(4):445–8.

14. Dzięgiel B, Adaszek Ł, Kalinowski M, et al. Equine granulocytic anaplasmosis. Res Vet Sci 2013;95(2):316–20.

15. Southwood LL, Schott HC, Henry CJ, et al. Disseminated hemangiosarcoma in the horse: 35 cases. J Vet Intern Med 2000;14:105–9.

16. Reef VB, Dyson SS, Beech J. Lymphosarcoma and associated immune-mediated hemolytic anemia and thrombocytopenia in horses. J Am Vet Med Assoc 1984; 184(3):313–7.

17. Hinchcliff KW, Kociba GJ, Mitten LA. Diagnosis of EDTA-dependent pseudo-thrombocytopenia in a horse. J Am Vet Med Assoc 1993;203:1715–6.

18. Barrell EA, Asakawa MG, Felippe MJB, et al. Acute leukemia in six horses (1990-2012). J Vet Diagn Invest 2017;29(4):529–35.

19. Bauer N, Nakagawa J, Dunker C, et al. Evaluation of the automated hematology analyzer Sysmex XT-2000iV ™ compared to the ADVIA ® 2120 for its use in dogs, cats, and horses. Part II: accuracy of leukocyte differential and reticulocyte count, impact of anticoagulant and sample aging. J Vet Diagn Invest 2012;24(1):74–89.

20. Blue JT, Dinsmore RP, Anderson KL. Immune-mediated hemolytic anemia induced by penicillin in horses. Cornell Vet 1987;77(3):263–76.

21. Cooper C, Sears W, Bienzle D. Reticulocyte changes after experimental anemia and erythropoietin treatment of horses. J Appl Physiol 2005;99:915–21.

22. Arnold CE, Chaffin MK. Abdominal abscesses in adult horses: 61 cases (1993-2008). J Am Vet Med Assoc 2012;241(12):1659–65.

23. Maxson AD, Reef VB. Bacterial endocarditis in horses: ten cases (1984-1995). Equine Vet J 1997;29(5):394–9.

24. Paulussen E, Lefère L, Bauwens C, et al. Yellow fat disease (steatitis) in 20 equids: description of clinical and ultrasonographic findings. Equine Vet Educ 2019;31(6):321–7.

25. Lavoie JP, Fiset L, Laverty S. Review of 40 cases of lung abscesses in foals and adult horses. Equine Vet J 1994;26(5):348–52.

26. Sellon DC, Levine JF, Palmer K, et al. Thrombocytosis in 24 horses (1989-1994). J Vet Intern Med 1997;11:24–9.

27. Alward A, Corriher CA, Barton MH, et al. Red maple (Acer rubrum) leaf toxicosis in horses: a retrospective study of 32 cases. J Vet Intern Med 2006;20:1197–201.

28. Thomas HL, Livesey MA. Immune-mediated hemolytic anemia associated with trimethroprim-sulphamethoxazole administration in a horse. Can Vet J 1998;39: 171–3.

29. Rose RJ, Allen JR, Hodgson DR, et al. Responses to submaximal treadmill exercise and training in the horse: changes in haematology, arterial blood gas and acid base measurements, plasma biochemical values and heart rate. Vet Rec 1983;113(26–27):612–8.

30. Jain NC. Hematology of the horse. In: Jain NC, editor. Schalm's veterinary hematology. 4th edition. Philadelphia: Lea & Febiger; 1986. p. 140–77.

31. Snow DH, Ricketts SW, Mason DK. Haematological response to racing and training exercise in Thoroughbred horses, with particular reference to the leucocyte response. Equine Vet J 1983;15(2):149–54.

32. Rodrigues A, Fighera RA, Souza TM, et al. Outbreaks of trypanosomiasis in horses by Trypanosoma evansi in the state of Rio Grande do Sul, Brazil: epidemiological, clinical, hematological, and pathological aspects. Pesqui Vet Bras 2005; 25(4):239–49.

33. Stannard AA, Gribble DH, Smith RS. Equine ehrlichiosis: a disease with similarities to tick-borne fever and bovine petechial fever. Vet Rec 1969;84(6):149–50.

34. Badial PR, Tallmadge RL, Miller S, et al. Applied protein and molecular techniques for characterization of B cell neoplasms in horses. Clin Vaccine Immunol 2015;22(11):1133–45.

35. Meyer J, Delay J, Bienzle D. Clinical, laboratory, and histopathologic features of equine lymphoma. Vet Pathol 2006;43:914–24.

36. Lumsden JH, Valli VEO, McSherry BJ. The comparison of erythrocyte and leukocyte response to epinephrine and acepromazine maleate in standardbred horses. Proc First Intern Symp Eq Haematol 1975;516–23.

37. Cooper CJ, Keller SM, Arroyo LG, et al. Acute Leukemia in Horses. Vet Pathol 2018;55(1):159–72.

38. Quist CF, Harmon BG, Mahaffey EA, et al. Large granular lymphocyte neoplasia in an aged mare. J Vet Diagn Invest 1994;6(1):111–3.

39. Meichner K, Kraszeski BH, Durrant JR, et al. Extreme lymphocytosis with myelomonocytic morphology in a horse with diffuse large B-cell lymphoma. Vet Clin Pathol 2017;46(1):64–71.

40. Harvey JW, Asquith RL, McNulty PK, et al. Haematology of foals up to one year old. Equine Vet J 1984;16(4):347–53.

41. Muñoz A, Riber C, Trigo P, et al. Age- and gender-related variations in hematology, clinical biochemistry, and hormones in Spanish fillies and colts. Res Vet Sci 2012;93(2):943–9.

42. Johnstone LK, Engiles JB, Aceto H, et al. Retrospective evaluation of horses diagnosed with neuroborreliosis on postmortem examination: 16 cases (2004-2015). J Vet Intern Med 2016;30(4):1305–12.

43. Wamsley HL, Alleman AR, Porter MB, et al. Cerebrospinal fluid findings in Florida horses with confirmed West Nile virus infection: 30 cases (2001). Vet Pathol 2002; 39:613.

44. Lester GD, Alleman AR, Raskin RE, et al. Pancytopenia secondary to lymphoid leukemia in three horses. J Vet Intern Med 1993;7:360–3.

45. Kelton DR, Holbrook TC, Gilliam LL, et al. Bone marrow necrosis and myelophthisis: manifestations of T-cell lymphoma in a horse. Vet Clin Pathol 2008;37:403–8.

46. Durando MM, Alleman AR, Harvey JW. Myelodysplastic syndrome in a Quarter Horse gelding. Equine Vet J 1994;26:83–5.

47. Lavoie JP, Morris DD, Zinkl JG, et al. Pancytopenia caused by bone marrow aplasia in a horse. J Am Vet Med Assoc 1987;191:1462–4.

48. Henry M, Prasse K, White S. Hemorrhagic diathesis caused by multiple myeloma in a three-month-old foal. J Am Vet Med Assoc 1989;194(3):392–4.

49. Angel KL, Spano JS, Schumacher J, et al. Myelophthisic pancytopenia in a pony mare. J Am Vet Med Assoc 1991;198:1039–42.

50. Tallmadge RL, Stokol T, Gould-Earley MJ, et al. Fell Pony syndrome: characterization of developmental hematopoiesis failure and associated gene expression profiles. Clin Vaccine Immunol 2012;19(7):1054–64.

51. Tvedten H, Riihimaki M. Hypersegmentation of equine neutrophils. Vet Clin Pathol 2007;36:4–5.

52. McFarlane D, Sellon DC, Parker B. Primary erythrocytosis in a 2-year-old Arabian gelding. J Vet Intern Med 1998;12:384–8.

53. Belli CB, Baccarin RY, Ida KK, et al. Appropriate secondary absolute erythrocytosis in a horse. Vet Rec 2011;169:609.

54. Cook G, Divers TJ, Rowland PH. Hypercalcemia and erythrocytosis in a mare associated with a metastatic carcinoma. Equine Vet J 1995;27:316–8.

55. Lavoie JP, Madigan JE, Cullor JS, et al. Haemodynamic, pathological, haematological and behavioural changes during endotoxin infusion in equine neonates. Equine Vet J 1990;22(1):23–9.

56. Targowski SP. Effect of prednisolone on the leukocyte counts of ponies and on the reactivity of lymphocytes in vitro and in vivo. Infect Immun 1975;11(2):252–6.

57. Rossdale PD, Burguez PN, Cash RS. Changes in blood neutrophil/lymphocyte ratio related to adrenocortical function in the horse. Equine Vet J 1982;14(4):293–8.

58. Boyle AG, Magdesian KG, Ruby RE. Neonatal isoerythrolysis in horse foals and a mule foal: 18 cases (1988-2003). J Am Vet Med Assoc 2005;227:1276–83.

59. Mair TS, Taylor FG, Hillyer MH. Autoimmune haemolytic anaemia in eight horses. Vet Rec 1990;126(3):51–3.

60. McGovern KF, Lascola KM, Davis E, et al. T-cell lymphoma with immune-mediated anemia and thrombocytopenia in a horse. J Vet Intern Med 2011; 25(5):1181–5.

61. Weiss DJ, Moritz A. Equine immune-mediated hemolytic anemia associated with Clostridium perfringens infection. Vet Clin Pathol 2003;32:22–6.

62. Reuss SM, Chaffin MK, Cohen ND. Extrapulmonary disorders associated with Rhodococcus equi infection in foals: 150 cases (1987-2007). J Am Vet Med Assoc 2009;235:855–63.

63. Bozorgmanesh R, Magdesian KG, Rhodes DM, et al. Hemolytic anemia in horses associated with ingestion of Pistacia leaves. J Vet Intern Med 2015;29(1):410–3.

64. Schott HC. Chronic renal failure in horses. Vet Clin North Am Equine Pract 2007; 23:593–612, vi.

65. Piercy RJ, Swardson CJ, Hinchcliff KW. Erythroid hypoplasia and anemia following administration of recombinant human erythropoietin to two horses. J Am Vet Med Assoc 1998;212:244–7.

66. Mastrorilli C, Cesar F, Joiner K, et al. Disseminated lymphoma with large granular lymphocyte morphology diagnosed in a horse via abdominal fluid and transtracheal wash cytology. Vet Clin Pathol 2015;44(3):437–41.

Bone Marrow Examination

Why, How, and What to Expect from the Pathologist

Dorothee Bienzle, DVM, PhD

KEYWORDS

- Anemia • Cytopenia • Equine • Horse • Leukopenia • Leukemia
- Myeloid neoplasia • Thrombocytopenia

KEY POINTS

- Tissue needs and bone marrow production of erythrocytes, leukocytes, and platelets are in a tightly controlled equilibrium.
- Persistent anemia, neutropenia, or thrombocytopenia that is unexplained by blood loss or systemic illness, or presence of morphologically abnormal cells on the blood smear are indications for examining marrow.
- Collection of marrow samples from sternebrae, and preparation of good-quality smears, requires expertise, caution, and some special equipment.
- Interpretation of marrow samples requires a concurrent complete blood cell count.
- Horses with acute leukemia are often overtly ill and have severe cytopenia and systemic inflammation.

OVERVIEW

The bone marrow produces red blood cells (RBC, erythrocytes), platelets, white blood cells (WBC, leukocytes), and precursors of lymphocytes. The number of new blood cells produced each day from hematopoietic precursor cells in mammals is enormous: approximately 100 billion each of erythrocytes, platelets, and neutrophils.[1–3] As such, the marrow is among the most mitotically active organs in the body. Once released from the marrow, erythrocytes, platelets, and neutrophils have relatively short circulation times of approximately 150 days, 10 days, and 8 hours, respectively.[4] Blood cells are removed from the circulation by the

Department of Pathobiology, University of Guelph, 50 Stone Road East, Guelph, Ontario N1G 2W1, Canada
E-mail address: dbienzle@uoguelph.ca

Vet Clin Equine 36 (2020) 35–52
https://doi.org/10.1016/j.cveq.2019.11.002
0749-0739/20/© 2019 Elsevier Inc. All rights reserved.

mononuclear phagocyte system (MPS) of the liver, spleen, and the marrow at a high rate because of aging (senescence), apoptosis, or exposure to oxidative and inflammatory stress. Components are catabolized for reuse and excretion. For example, iron from erythrocytes is returned to marrow and spleen for storage and reuse, whereas heme is broken down to bilirubin for disposal via the gastrointestinal and urinary tract. Production of blood cells by the marrow and removal by the MPS is a very dynamic and tightly regulated process, which translates to tight limits for the number of each cell type that is in circulation during health. In turn, this fine regulation of blood cells is used to establish meaningful reference intervals for complete blood cell counts (CBC). On the other hand, the marrow has tremendous capacity to increase the production of all hematopoietic cells. The latter is illustrated by conditions such as immune-mediated anemia or thrombocytopenia, whereby the lifespan of RBC and platelets may be reduced to hours, and in turn, marrow output increases many times over. Similarly, in bacterial diseases with extensive tissue inflammation, such as Potomac horse fever caused by *Neorickettsia risticii* or salmonellosis, neutrophils accumulate rapidly in large numbers in the inflamed colon, which causes neutropenia and stimulates marrow granulopoiesis. Often horses that recover subsequently have transient neutrophilia.[5] As such, blood and marrow form a single contiguous organ the adequacy of which can be assessed with a CBC, and unexplained abnormalities on the CBC can be investigated with marrow biopsy.

LYMPHOCYTES

Lymphocytes normally encompass 20% to 50% of circulating leukocytes in horses. They are long lived and only traverse briefly in and out of the vasculature as they travel between lymph nodes, spleen, and lymphoid niches in other organs, such as the intestine, liver, and skin. Lymphocyte stem cells originate in marrow, and aged plasma cells return to marrow, but their predominant location and turnover are in lymphoid tissues. The marrow of mature horses normally harbors only a few lymphocytes (<5%–10% of nucleated cells). Furthermore, lymphocytes in circulation represent only a minor fraction of the total body lymphocytes and reflect overall immune reactivity rather than marrow function. As a result, lymphopenia is most often associated with active immune responses and retention of lymphocytes in lymphoid tissues. Foals in the first week of life are normally lymphopenic relative to adult horses, and then lymphocyte numbers progressively increase to reach those of adult horses by 2 to 3 weeks of age.[6,7] Persistent and severe lymphopenia may indicate a generalized immune deficiency, such as severe combined immunodeficiency. Different phases and types of inflammation, and acute viral infections, may be associated with mild or transient lymphopenia or lymphocytosis, and altered lymphocyte morphologic features, such as increased size and cytoplasmic basophilia.[8] In adult thoroughbred horses, exercise caused a transient lymphocytosis, whereas administration of adrenocorticotrophic hormone caused neutrophilia and a mild lymphopenia.[9] Lymphopenia was observed after exercise and in association with increased plasma catecholamine concentration.[10] Overall, alterations in blood lymphocyte numbers rarely persist outside the reference interval, consistent with the small and dynamic contribution of circulating lymphocytes to total body lymphocytes. Corresponding to their benign counterparts, lymphocytic leukemias in the marrow are either acute poorly differentiated (acute lymphocytic leukemia, ALL) or terminally differentiated types (chronic lymphocytic leukemia, CLL).

INDICATORS OF BONE MARROW DISEASE

Failure of the marrow to produce adequate hematopoietic precursors causes anemia, neutropenia, and/or thrombocytopenia. Horses with anemia have pale mucous membranes and often exercise intolerance. The effects of neutropenia are opportunistic infections, fever, and malaise, and lack of platelets renders horses prone to bleeding. The degree of cytopenia and the rapidity of onset contribute to the severity of clinical signs. For example, spontaneous epistaxis does not usually occur until the platelet count is less than 20,000 to 50,000/μL (most laboratories have horse platelet reference intervals of approximately 100,000–400,000/μL), although effective platelet function is also influenced by the size and age of the platelets. The following is a suggested approach to horses with cytopenia in order to decide if a marrow biopsy is needed:

1. *Complete physical examination.* Assess the horse for the color of mucous membranes, dehydration, presence of edema, sites of inflammation, fever, and enlarged lymph nodes. Query the owner regarding food intake, weight loss, occurrence of diarrhea, past treatments, vaccination, and anthelminthic therapy. Acute systemic bacterial infections, such as salmonellosis or Potomac horse fever, frequently cause neutropenia with a left shift, but also manifest with acute diarrhea.[5,11] Endotoxemia injures neutrophil precursors in marrow, and experimental administration caused severe neutropenia within minutes followed by neutrophilia after 8 hours.[12] Experimental infection with *Anaplasma phagocytophilum* caused mild transient anemia and leukopenia, and moderate thrombocytopenia in addition to anorexia, pyrexia, and edema, and similar findings were reported in naturally occurring infections.[13–15] Edema owing to hypoalbuminemia and lymphatic obstruction from enlarged lymph nodes is a common feature of lymphoma in horses, but hypoalbuminemia can also result from gastrointestinal parasitism, *Lawsonia intracellularis* infection, malnutrition, and other causes.[16–18] Horses with lymphocytic and myeloid leukemia may also have enlarged lymph nodes.[19,20]

2. *Verify the CBC abnormalities.* In-house hematology analyzers are generally not subject to as extensive a quality-assurance and quality-control program as those in reference laboratories and do not generate as much detail. Therefore, in horses with abnormal findings on a CBC, the analysis should be repeated in a reference laboratory to confirm persistence and nature of the hematologic abnormality.

3. *Review the numerical CBC indices.* Advanced hematology analyzers interrogate thousands of blood cells for a CBC and generate powerful statistical information in addition to determining the standard parameters of hematocrit (HCT), hemoglobin concentration, WBC, and platelet number. For example, the red cell distribution width (RDW) is a useful indicator of the degree of RBC anisocytosis, which can reflect marrow erythropoietic activity. In regenerative anemia, increases in RDW precede increases in mean cell volume (MCV), and both indices may be used to gauge the duration of anemia and extent of marrow response.[21,22] Additional potentially useful numerical indices are platelet volume and plateletcrit (PCT). Similar to RBC, platelets recently released from marrow can be larger than those that have circulated for

days, and a large mean platelet volume (MPV) can indicate increased thrombopoiesis. The PCT accounts for both the number of platelets and their size. Of note, samples that are not analyzed fresh but rather stored for 24 or 48 hours at refrigeration can show increases in MPV and platelet number because of cell swelling and fragmentation.[23] In-practice and reference hematology analyzers generally determine the total WBC count accurately, but automated differential counts may be inaccurate in samples from diseased horses.[24] In acute inflammation, neutropenia results from rapidly induced adhesion of neutrophils to venous walls and subsequent exit from the vasculature into tissues. Increased production of new neutrophils takes several days; therefore, acute inflammation is typically associated with transient neutropenia and a left shift. Primary marrow diseases, such as leukemia, cause neutropenia owing to myelophthisis or suppression of normal hematopoiesis.[19,20]

4. *Evaluate a blood smear.* A blood smear prepared from fresh EDTA anticoagulated blood should be assessed for the following:
   a. RBC agglutination: This occurs in many cases of lymphoma and leukemia, but can also occur in bacterial (*Streptococcus* spp, *Clostridium* spp) infection, acute equine infectious anemia virus infection, and secondary to antimicrobial treatment.
   b. Intravascular hemolysis: All of the above conditions may cause agglutination in conjunction with RBC lysis, as indicated by RBC ghosts on the blood smear.
   c. Infectious agents: *Theileria equi* and *Babesia caballi* are piroplasms that infect RBC and cause extravascular hemolysis but not usually agglutination. The organisms may be seen on blood smears during acute infection.[25]
   d. Leukocyte morphology: A manual differential leukocyte count should be performed and compared with that generated by the automated analyzer. Bacterial infections are often associated with a left shift in neutrophils, indicating release of immature neutrophils in response to overwhelming tissue demand. Depending on the magnitude of the tissue demand, there may be concurrent neutropenia. Neutrophils released from marrow under stress conditions often contain basophilic cytoplasmic aggregates termed Döhle bodies and have poorly segmented nuclei (**Fig. 1**A). Immature cells, blasts, and cells that cannot be classified as normal leukocytes (**Fig. 1**B) should be enumerated separately.
   e. Erythrocyte morphology: Release of rubricytes (nucleated RBC) from marrow is abnormal and extremely rare in horses (**Fig. 1**C). Automated instruments do not detect rubricytes. Rubricytes have rarely been reported in any condition other than leukemia.[19,20,26]
   f. Absence of platelet clumps: Artifactual thrombocytopenia from platelets that are aggregated because of inadequate anticoagulation should be ruled out by evaluating the blood film for clumps. Platelet clumping may occur because of inadequate blood anticoagulation or collection of samples from catheters.

The above steps will maximize information gleaned from thorough hematological analysis. If repeated CBC confirms persistent cytopenia, cytosis, or presence of atypical cells, and if infectious and toxic causes have been ruled out, a core biopsy and marrow aspirate should be obtained.

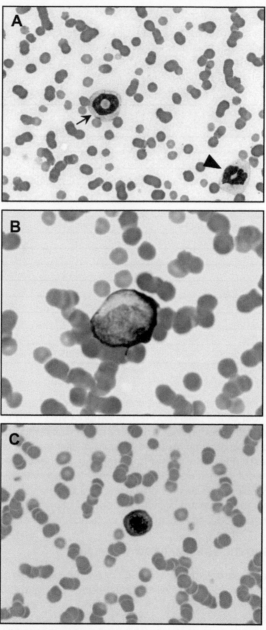

Fig. 1. (A) Blood film from a gelding with salmonellosis and neutropenia. There are toxic changes in neutrophils and a left shift as illustrated by the band neutrophil with a circular nucleus ("donut"; *arrow*) and cytoplasmic basophilia (*arrowhead*); ×60 objective. (B) A very large blast (approximately 30 μm in diameter) in the blood film of a 9-year-old thoroughbred mare with marked anemia, neutropenia, and thrombocytopenia of more than 2 weeks' duration, and a subsequent diagnosis of AML; ×100 objective. (C) Rubricyte in the same blood film as in panel B; ×60 objective. All blood films were prepared with Wright stain.

CASE 1

A thoroughbred-Welsh cross mare, 3 years old and used as a riding horse, had poor appetite and 2 episodes of epistaxis in the last week. Results of an in-practice CBC indicated anemia and thrombocytopenia. The horse was referred, and the CBC was repeated with the following results:

Parameter	Result	Unit	Reference Interval
WBC	4.5 L	×10⁹/L	5.1–11.0
RBC	5.1 L	×10¹²/L	6.9–10.7
Hemoglobin	78 L	g/L	112–169
HCT	0.22 L	L/L	0.38–0.55
MCV	44	fL	42–53
Mean corpuscular hemoglobin (MCH)	15	pg	14–18
Mean corpuscular hemoglobin concentration (MCHC)	351	g/L	324–354
RDW	18.9	%	16.3–20.4
Platelets	44 L	×10⁹/L	83–270
MPV	8.2	fL	6–11
Neutrophils	0.14 L	×10⁹/L	2.8–7.7
Lymphocytes	4.19	×10⁹/L	1.3–4.7
Monocytes	0.14	×10⁹/L	0.1–0.8
Rubricytes	0.05 H	×10⁹/L	0

Review of the blood smear confirmed anemia, thrombocytopenia, and neutropenia and showed that most of the cells reported as lymphocytes were very large (**Fig. 2**A). Serum biochemical evaluation indicated low urea, creatinine, and bilirubin concentrations. A marrow core and aspirate revealed a highly cellular marrow consisting predominantly of large blasts (**Fig. 2**B–D). The presumptive diagnosis was ALL, which was confirmed with phenotyping tests. The horse was treated with glucocorticoids and euthanized after 6 weeks because of anorexia and clinical deterioration. On postmortem examination, the horse had ventral skin and duodenal petechiation, gastric ulceration, and distortion of lymph node, spleen, and liver architecture by neoplastic lymphocytes.

COLLECTING DIAGNOSTIC BONE MARROW SAMPLES

Over the past decade, sampling of marrow in horses has become more commonplace because of the demand for stem cell therapies, and several detailed protocols are available.[27,28] In adult horses, active or red marrow is concentrated in cancellous bones that contain trabeculae, and therefore, a large surface area for hematopoiesis that is in intimate contact with bone and adipose tissue. Practically, the most accessible locations for bone marrow biopsy in horses are the sternebrae because they can be reached with a 10-cm Jamshidi needle, and because the cortex of the sternebra is thinner than that of the pelvis or long bones.

The following steps maximize the likelihood of obtaining a diagnostic combined marrow core biopsy and aspirate from the sternum of a horse:

1. Assemble at least 1 assistant, clippers, materials for aseptic skin preparation, 23-gauge hypodermic needles, 3-mL and 12-mL syringes, local anesthetic, scalpel

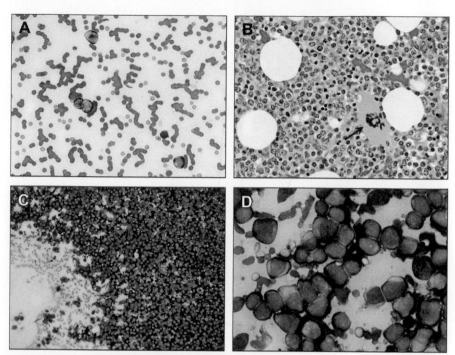

Fig. 2. Samples from a 3-year-old mare with anemia, neutropenia, and thrombocytopenia (case 1). (*A*) The blood film shows reduced RBC density (anemia), absence of neutrophils, and predominance of blasts; ×40 objective, Wright stain. (*B*) On histopathology, the marrow consists predominantly of large blasts with round nuclei. There are no segmented neutrophils, and only rare rubricytes and 1 megakaryocyte (*arrow*); ×40 objective, hematoxylin and eosin stain. (*C*) The marrow aspirate is highly cellular and almost exclusively composed of blasts; ×20 objective, Wright stain. (*D*) At high magnification, the marrow blasts are 20 to 30 μm in diameter and have round to slightly angular nuclei. The diagnosis was ALL, based on additional phenotyping tests; ×60 objective, Wright stain.

blades, a sterile 11-gauge/10-cm (4-in) Jamshidi needle, 1 to 2 mL of sterile 1% EDTA solution or citrate aspirated from a blood transfusion bag, 8 to 10 glass slides, absorbent paper towels, a jar of B5 fixative or 10% buffered formalin, and gauze. Jamshidi needles have a trocar fitting the lumen of the needle to protect the sharp tip of the needle as it moves through cortical bone, are slightly tapered toward the tip to assist with retention of the core, and come with a flat-ended probe for retrograde dislodgement of the core.

2. Place the horse in stocks and sedate. Although marrow aspiration itself in sedated horses has been considered minimally painful, a stab skin incision is required, and the operator has to locate below the horse's chest.[29] Therefore, the horse should be adequately sedated to assure safety for the operator, even for mild-mannered horses.

3. Clip and surgically prepare the skin overlying the sternum. The fifth and sixth sternebrae are most suitable for marrow aspiration because of proximity to the ventral skin, distinct intersternebral cartilaginous spaces, and adequate dorso-ventral distance (**Fig. 3**). The seventh sternebra is proximal to the apex of the heart and may be partially fused with the sixth sternebra and should therefore be avoided. Sternebrae and intersternebral spaces may be visualized with

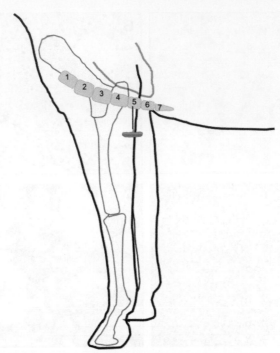

Fig. 3. Diagram of approximate location of sternebrae and placement of a bone marrow biopsy needle (*blue*). Location of the heart is indicated by the red line.

ultrasound, but, in general, the fourth sternebra is slightly cranial to the olecranon, and the fifth sternebra is at a line drawn between the olecranons. Of particular importance is that the horse stands square with front legs at a similar angle, and that all needle entries are exactly on the anterior-posterior midline and perpendicular to the surface of the skin. A detailed description of the location and accessibility of sternebrae for marrow aspiration is provided by Kasashima and colleagues.[27]

4. Infiltrate the skin, subcutaneous tissue, and periosteum with 2 to 5 mL of 2% lidocaine. A 3.75-cm (1.5 in) hypodermic needle will just reach the sternebral cortex in a horse of average size, and no further advancement should be possible.

5. Apply a final aseptic skin cleansing. Make a stab incision with a size 11 scalpel blade in a sterile fashion at the site of prior local anesthetic infiltration. Insert the sterile Jamshidi needle with the trochar in place and gradually advance through the subcutaneous tissue. Keep the needle perpendicular to the skin and do not deviate. Once the periosteum has been reached, slowly advance the needle by rotating with moderate pressure and continue to maintain a perpendicular orientation.

6. Once the needle is seated in cortical bone and feels firmly in place, remove the trochar and place it on a sterile surface. Advance the hollow needle for 2 to 3 cm (most Jamshidi needles have 1-cm graduation rings on the outside of the needle to assist with gauging the depth) to "cut" a cylinder of trabecular bone marrow. Rotate the needle in an attempt to break off the distal part of the marrow cylinder. Retract the needle 2 to 3 mm and advance again at a slight angle to help with transecting the distal end of the core. Retract the needle and exit through the skin.

7. Apply gauze to the skin if there is more than slight hemorrhage. Feed the flat-ended probe into the tip of the Jamshidi needle and push out the core in a

retrograde manner. A fresh nonfixed core should be at least 2 cm in length and is normally red. Place the core into the fixative. If the core is less than 2 cm long, repeat the procedure.

8. Maintaining sterility, rinse the needle with ~1 mL of sterile EDTA or citrate, reassemble the trocar into the Jamshidi needle, and place the needle as above in the bone marrow cavity. The same path as for the core biopsy may be followed. Once the needle is again seated firmly in bone, remove the trocar and attach a 12-mL syringe. Aspirate vigorously until the syringe contains 0.5 to 1 mL of marrow. Aspirated marrow has an appearance of thick blood with flecks of fat.

9. Remove the syringe and needle, detach the syringe, and quickly prepare slides. Place a thick drop of marrow toward the frosted edge of 4 to 6 glass slides. Tilt the slides sideways to let the blood run off onto absorbent paper. Marrow spicules will adhere to glass. Prepare a minimum of 2, and ideally up to 4 to 10, each of squash and feathered edge–type smears (**Fig. 4**). Dry the slides quickly by waving in the air or placing in front of a fan or hairdryer.

10. Apply pressure to the site of skin penetration or a temporary surcingle bandage with sterile gauze and an elastic bandage to stop bleeding.

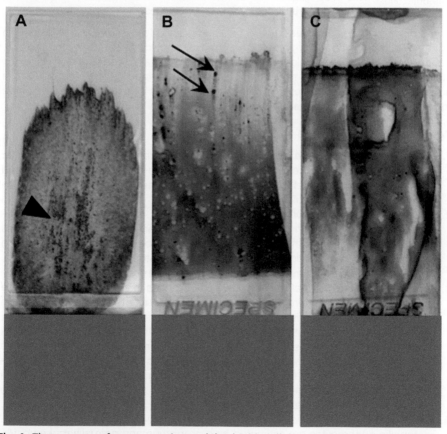

Fig. 4. Three smears of marrow aspirates. (*A*) A highly cellular squash preparation with particles spread apart (*arrowhead*). (*B*) A moderately cellular "feather-edge" preparation with small intact particles near the edge (*arrows*). (*C*) A poorly cellular aspirate devoid of marrow particles. All slides were Wright stained.

Additional Tips

- It is essential to obtain the core biopsy before aspirating. Aspirating marrow induces sinusoidal rupture and therefore hemorrhage, disrupts marrow architecture, and compromises subsequent histologic evaluation of core sections.
- It takes longer to collect both a core and an aspirate, but the equipment and sampling approach are the same, and having both types of sample yields much more information than either one alone.
- Marrow clots quickly; therefore, rinsing the Jamshidi needle and the syringe with 0.5 to 1 mL of sterile 1% EDTA solution or citrate aspirated from a blood transfusion bag before aspiration or retained in the syringe is helpful. Once anticoagulated, the marrow aspirate can also be placed into a Petri dish, and particles can be harvested with a glass pipette for making less bloody high-quality smears. Without anticoagulant, slides have to be prepared very quickly.
- Sterile technique is particularly important in neutropenic horses.
- Thrombocytopenia is generally not a contraindication to marrow biopsy. The bone marrow cavity is an enclosed space that contains bleeding.
- For diagnostic purposes, the first 0.5 to 1 mL of a marrow aspirate is best and sufficient. This initial aliquot has far more cells than subsequent aliquots that are diluted with blood from ruptured marrow sinuses.[28]

Interpreting marrow samples can be challenging, and ideally, a pathologist versed in both cytopathology and histopathology of marrow should assess both preparations. Because hematopoiesis is highly dynamic, and blood cells represent the marrow's output, it is essential that all marrow samples be interpreted in conjunction with the horse's history and concurrent hematological findings. Therefore, a blood sample for a CBC should be submitted together with the marrow samples.

WHAT TO EXPECT FROM THE PATHOLOGIST'S REPORT

1. *Comment on whether the sample quantity and quality are adequate.* Cytologic preparations should be cellular, thin to assure single-cell distribution, and dried quickly to preserve cell detail. Core biopsies should have a minimum of 3 intertrabecular spaces free of artifact.
2. *Indication of the presence of particles and their cellularity, the frequency of megakaryocytes, and adequacy of iron stores.* Good-quality marrow smears from healthy horses have 5 to 10 particles, and the particles are 30% to 70% cellular, with lower cellularity in advancing age. There should be 3 to 6 megakaryocytes associated with each particle, and in adult horses, iron stores should be readily apparent in each particle.
3. *Description of whether maturation in all 3 cell lineages is synchronous or not, and whether dysplastic cells are present.* A differential count of 500 cells on cytologic smears is helpful to objectively enumerate cell types and will indicate the proportion of blasts. The granulocytic-to-erythrocytic (G/E) ratio, also called myeloid-to-erythroid ratio, in horses is normally 1:1 to 1:2.5, meaning erythrocytic precursors are normally equal to more frequent than granulocytic precursors. Maturing, nonproliferating granulocytes (metamyelocytes, band neutrophils, segmented neutrophils) normally outnumber immature, proliferating granulocytes (myeloblasts, promyelocytes, myelocytes) by greater than 3:1.
4. *Comment on the proportion of polychromatophilic erythrocytes.* These polychromatophilic erythrocytes are estimated as a proportion and normally make up 1% to 2% of erythrocytes.
5. *Presence of myelofibrosis, necrosis, gelatinous transformation of fat, and nonuniform distribution of hematopoiesis is best assessed on histologic sections.*

The marrow report should consider whether there is an appropriate response to a systemic condition. Examples include the following:

- With chronic or severe blood loss leading to anemia, the marrow should have greater than 70% erythropoietic precursors; the G/E should be less than 1:3 and could be as low as 1:5, and polychromatophilic erythrocytes should be greater than 2%.[22]
- Long-term treatment of horses with erythropoietin may lead to erythrocytosis and an increased proportion of rubricytes in marrow.[21] In rare cases of lymphoma, there may be paraneoplastic production of erythropoietin, also leading to erythrocytosis and increased marrow rubricytes.[30]
- Chronic neutrophilic inflammation from conditions such as dermatitis will induce hyperplasia of granulocytic precursor cells and may shift the G/E from 1:2 to greater than 3:1.
- Immune-mediated thrombocytopenia may relapse after treatment and may result in megakaryocytic hyperplasia with greater than 10 megakaryocytes per particle.[31]
- Malnutrition and cachexia may induce gelatinous transformation of marrow fat ("serous" atrophy of fat), which in turn affects hematopoiesis, leading to cytopenia. This has been described in a miniature horse with severe dental disease[32] and may be more frequent in areas with endemic poor nutrition.
- In general, cytopenia that persists for more than 2 weeks without an identified cause, such as hemorrhage, inflammation, or iron deficiency, is most often associated with primary marrow disease, such as leukemia.

TYPES OF LEUKEMIA

Neoplasms of hematopoietic cells (leukemias) are broadly divided into myeloid and lymphoid types and further classified, based on the duration and severity of cytopenia and the number of blasts, into acute and chronic forms. Features typical of different types of leukemia include the following.

Acute Myeloid Leukemia

- Affected horses have severe and usually multiple and severe cytopenia, vague illness (hyporexia, intermittent fever, lethargy) for a few days to a few weeks, and signs of systemic inflammation, such as increases in the acute phase proteins fibrinogen, serum amyloid A or haptoglobin, hyperglobulinemia, and RBC may be agglutinating.
- Lack of a leukocytosis, sometimes termed "subleukemia" or "aleukemic leukemia," is typical of acute myeloid leukemia (AML) in horses.[19,20,33]
- Concentrating leukocytes with buffy coat preparations may reveal morphologically abnormal cells.
- Marrow aspirates range from normocellular to hypercellular and have greater than 20% blasts.
- In most cases of AML, there is no entirely predominant cell population (such as myeloblasts), but various stages of rubricytes and some differentiated granulocytes are present, in addition to greater than 30% blasts.
- The diagnosis of AML hinges on the presence of an increased proportion of blasts, lack of synchronous maturation of granulocytes, rubricytes, or megakaryocytes, combined with severe cytopenias and/or the presence of blasts in peripheral blood.
- Myelomonocytic differentiation (leukemic cells have features of both neutrophils and monocytes) was most common among 25 to 30 reported cases of equine AML.[19,20,34–39]

- In some forms of AML, the predominant population of blasts and immature granulocytes may belong to the eosinophil or basophil lineages.[20]
- Basophil AML may be associated with otherwise unexplained failure of hemostasis.[20]

Acute Lymphocytic Leukemia

- As with AML, horses with ALL also often have signs of systemic inflammation and a history of intermittent fever, hyporexia, and lethargy.
- Horses with ALL are generally younger than 4 years of age, whereas the age of horses with AML can range from young to geriatric.
- Cytopenias are usually as severe in ALL as in AML, but enlargement of lymph nodes and splenomegaly may be more common in ALL.
- Marrow samples are more uniformly composed of neoplastic large lymphocytes (see **Fig. 2**) than the proportion of myeloblasts present in AML (**Fig. 5**).
- Immunohistochemistry or flow cytometry can be used to classify ALL into B- or T-cell type, but no prognostic differences between different types of ALL have been shown.
- Some cases of equine lymphoma have extensive marrow involvement and many circulating neoplastic lymphocytes; therefore, distinguishing between ALL and lymphoma may not be unequivocal.[17,40]

Biologically, leukemic cells have clonal somatic mutations, and predominance of a particular morphologic type results from mutations in specific cytokine receptors, signaling molecules, or transcription factors that favor development or arrest of that cell type.[41] Some acute leukemia cases in horses have features of both AML and ALL (mixed lymphoid/myeloid phenotype), and distinguishing the neoplastic population from an inflammatory component based on morphology may be challenging.[42] The prognosis for horses with either AML or ALL is uniformly poor. Combination chemotherapy was unsuccessfully tried in 1 case, but most horses, whether treated with glucocorticoids or not, survived only a few days to weeks after diagnosis.[19,20,33] Postmortem evaluation can reveal extramedullary leukemic lesions on serosal surfaces and multiple organs.[19,20]

Chronic Lymphocytic Leukemia

Chronic types of leukemia also occur in horses, but appear to be less common than acute leukemias with only 1 reported small case series.[43] The clinicopathologic features of chronic leukemia in general are a cytosis of neoplastic cells that are morphologically similar to their benign counterpart, with concurrent cytopenia involving only 1 cell line and/or of milder degree and/or longer duration than cytopenias in acute leukemia. The lymphocytosis may be discovered incidentally or owing to investigation of exercise intolerance. Horses with CLL were older and had marked lymphocytosis and often mild neutropenia or anemia.[42–46] In all cases, the lymphocyte count increased over a few weeks or months, despite 1 horse having been treated with prednisolone and chlorambucil.[45] Hyperglobulinemia was noted in most horses, and also in case 2 described in later discussion. Enlargement of lymph nodes and edema were common at the time of diagnosis, and organ infiltration by neoplastic lymphocytes was noted in cases that underwent postmortem evaluation.[42–46] Overall, CLL appears to be relatively uncommon in horses, and diagnosis does not necessarily require marrow assessment.

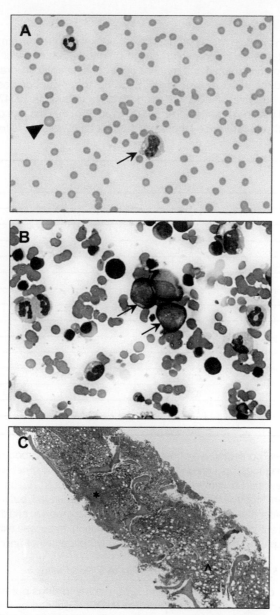

Fig. 5. Samples from a 21-year-old thoroughbred mare with anemia, neutropenia, and thrombocytopenia. (*A*) The blood film shows reduced RBC density, large erythrocytes (*arrowhead*), and absence of platelets. Atypical large cells with features of both monocytes and neutrophils (*arrow*) comprising 47% of the differential leukocyte count; ×40 objective, Wright stain. (*B*) The bone marrow aspirate has 21% blasts (*arrows*) and only rare polychromatophilic cells; ×60 objective, Wright stain. (*C*) The core biopsy has minimal artifact and greater than 5 intertrabecular spaces. Overall cellularity is approximately 90%, but there are 100% cellular areas (*asterisk*) and other areas with interspersed adipose cells of 60% to 70% cellularity (*circ*). Therefore, hematopoiesis is nonuniform, which is abnormal. Megakaryocytes are rare. The diagnosis was AML, and the horse was euthanized because of rapid clinical deterioration; ×10 objective, hematoxylin and eosin stain.

CASE 2

An 18-year old Clydesdale mare had hyporexia, brisket, ventral abdominal, distal limb and periorbital edema, and mildly enlarged lymph nodes. Serum biochemical analysis showed mild hypoalbuminemia and marked hyperglobulinemia. In-practice CBC indicated marked leukocytosis of 132 × 10^9/L owing to a lymphocytosis, low normal neutrophil count, anemia of 0.18 L/L, and thrombocytopenia of 47 × 10^9/L. The mare was treated with dexamethasone and referred (**Fig. 6**). Findings on the CBC performed at the author's reference laboratory 1 week later were as follows:

Parameter	Result	Unit	Reference Interval
WBC	85.5 H	×10^9/L	5.1–11.0
RBC	3.1 L	×10^{12}/L	6.9–10.7
Hemoglobin	58 L	g/L	112–169
HCT	0.17 L	L/L	0.38–0.55
MCV	53	fL	42–53
MCH	17	pg	14–18
MCHC	340	g/L	324–354
RDW	18.1	%	16.3–20.4
Platelets	69 L	×10^9/L	83–270
MPV	9.3	fL	6–11
Neutrophils	1.24 L	×10^9/L	2.8–7.7
Band neutrophils	0.85 H	×10^9/L	0.0–0.2
Lymphocytes	82.27 H	×10^9/L	1.3–4.7
Monocytes	1.14 H	×10^9/L	0.1–0.8
Eosinophils	0	×10^9/L	0.0–0.7

Blood film review confirmed lymphocytosis, anemia, and thrombocytopenia and also showed a proteinaceous background consistent with hyperglobulinemia. Serum protein electrophoresis revealed a narrow peak in the gamma-globulin region, suggestive of a monoclonal protein. Treatment with dexamethasone was continued, but the lymphocytosis progressed to greater than 150 × 10^9/L over the subsequent month, and the horse became anorexic and was euthanized. On postmortem examination, there was extensive infiltration of marrow, liver, spleen, and lymph nodes by small lymphocytes of uniform morphology.

Myelodysplastic Syndrome and Myeloproliferative Neoplasm

These neoplastic disorders are recognized in humans and dogs but are not well characterized in horses. Myelodysplastic syndrome (MDS) is defined by mild and gradually progressive cytopenias, marrow hyperplasia, blast counts between 5% and 20%, and dysplasia in greater than 10% of blood or marrow cells.[47] Affected patients have variably rapid progression of disease with eventual failure of hematopoiesis and/or progression to AML. Cases of MDS in horses meeting these criteria have not been reported, although dysplasia can be a feature of AML.[20,48] Myeloproliferative neoplasms (MPN) are chronic nonlymphocytic leukemias that in humans and small animals manifest with marked cytosis of neutrophils, eosinophils, monocytes, erythrocytes, or platelets. Although a case of chronic granulocytic leukemia in a horse was reported, the individual had a moderate leukocytosis, and a severe anemia and thrombocytopenia, which would be consistent with criteria for AML rather than MPN.[26]

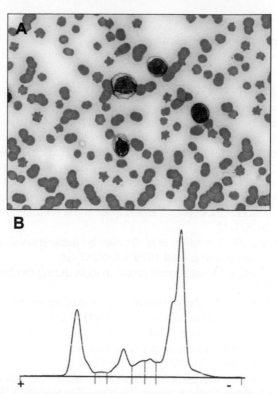

Fig. 6. Samples from an 18-year-old Clydesdale mare with lymphocytosis, thrombocyto-penia, and hyperglobulinemia (case 2). (*A*) The lymphocytes are of small to medium size (approximately 20 μm in diameter) and have pale blue cytoplasm. The background of the film is bluish, which suggests hyperproteinemia; ×40 objective, Wright stain. (*B*) Serum pro-tein electrophoresis identifies a small albumin peak (anode, +) and a tall and narrow peak in the gamma-globulin region (cathode, −), suggestive of a clonal immunoglobulin. The diagnosis was CLL.

Multiple Myeloma

Multiple myeloma is a neoplasm of plasma cells that has been reported in horses.[49,50] The marrow and other tissues are infiltrated by clusters of plasma cells, which may result in cytopenia owing to hematopoiesis-suppressing factors elaborated by tumor cells, and myelophthisis. Marrow biopsy is not usually needed to diagnose multiple myeloma because hyperglobulinemia and detection of clonal globulins on electropho-resis of urine or serum samples are specific and noninvasive diagnostic steps. In some cases of lymphoma and CLL, neoplastic B cells may also produce clonal immunoglobulins.[17]

In summary, the need for bone marrow biopsy arises from unexplained and persis-tent hematological abnormalities. Interpretation of samples should first rule out whether marrow findings are in response to benign conditions such as chronic hem-orrhage or inflammation. If leukemia is diagnosed, classification as AML or ALL should be attempted. Horses with acute leukemia have severe cytopenia, rapid disease pro-gression, and poor or no response to therapy. Distinction between ALL and AML is not always feasible. Chronic leukemia of either lymphoid or myeloid type is rare, and MDS akin to the disease in other species has not been reported in horses.

DISCLOSURE

There was no funding for this review article.

REFERENCES

1. Summers C, Rankin SM, Condliffe AM, et al. Neutrophil kinetics in health and disease. Trends Immunol 2010;31(8):318–24.
2. Qadri SM, Bissinger R, Solh Z, et al. Eryptosis in health and disease: a paradigm shift towards understanding the (patho)physiological implications of programmed cell death of erythrocytes. Blood Rev 2017;31(6):349–61.
3. Grozovsky R, Giannini S, Falet H, et al. Novel mechanisms of platelet clearance and thrombopoietin regulation. Curr Opin Hematol 2015;22(5):445–51.
4. Carter EI, Valli VE, McSherry BJ, et al. The kinetics of hematopoiesis in the light horse. I. The lifespan of peripheral blood cells in the normal horse. Can J Comp Med 1974;38(3):303–13.
5. Owen R, Fullerton JN, Tizard IR, et al. Studies on experimental enteric salmonellosis in ponies. Can J Comp Med 1979;43(3):247–54.
6. Faramarzi B, Rich L. Haematological profile in foals during the first year of life. Vet Rec 2019;184(16):503.
7. Lumsden JH, Rowe R, Mullen K. Hematology and biochemistry reference values for the light horse. Can J Comp Med 1980;44(1):32–42.
8. Brault SA, Blanchard MT, Gardner IA, et al. The immune response of foals to natural infection with equid herpesvirus-2 and its association with febrile illness. Vet Immunol Immunopathol 2010;137(1–2):136–41.
9. Rossdale PD, Burguez PN, Cash RS. Changes in blood neutrophil/lymphocyte ratio related to adrenocortical function in the horse. Equine Vet J 1982;14(4):293–8.
10. Cuniberti B, Badino P, Odore R, et al. Effects induced by exercise on lymphocyte β-adrenergic receptors and plasma catecholamine levels in performance horses. Res Vet Sci 2012;92(1):116–20.
11. Bertin FR, Reising A, Slovis NM, et al. Clinical and clinicopathological factors associated with survival in 44 horses with equine neorickettsiosis (Potomac horse fever). J Vet Intern Med 2013;27(6):1528–34.
12. Lilliehöök I, Tvedten HW, Bröjer J, et al. Time-related changes in equine neutrophils after experimental endotoxemia: myeloperoxidase staining, size, and numbers. Vet Clin Pathol 2016;45(1):66–72.
13. Davies RS, Madigan JE, Hodzic E, et al. Dexamethasone-induced cytokine changes associated with diminished disease severity in horses infected with Anaplasma phagocytophilum. Clin Vaccine Immunol 2011;18(11):1962–8.
14. Franzén P, Aspan A, Egenvall A, et al. Acute clinical, hematologic, serologic, and polymerase chain reaction findings in horses experimentally infected with a European strain of Anaplasma phagocytophilum. J Vet Intern Med 2005;19(2):232–9.
15. Jahn P, Zeman P, Bezdekova B, et al. Equine granulocytic anaplasmosis in the Czech Republic. Vet Rec 2010;166(21):646–9.
16. Durham AC, Pillitteri CA, San Myint M, et al. Two hundred three cases of equine lymphoma classified according to the World Health Organization (WHO) classification criteria. Vet Pathol 2013;50(1):86–93.
17. Meyer J, DeLay J, Bienzle D. Clinical, laboratory, and histopathologic features of equine lymphoma. Vet Pathol 2006;43(6):914–24.
18. Peregrine AS, McEwen B, Bienzle D, et al. Larval cyathostominosis in horses in Ontario: an emerging disease? Can Vet J 2006;47(1):80–2.

19. Barrell EA, Asakawa MG, Felippe MJB, et al. Acute leukemia in six horses (1990-2012). J Vet Diagn Invest 2017;29(4):529–35.
20. Cooper CJ, Keller SM, Arroyo LG, et al. Acute leukemia in horses. Vet Pathol 2018;55(1):159–72.
21. Cooper C, Sears W, Bienzle D. Reticulocyte changes after experimental anemia and erythropoietin treatment of horses. J Appl Physiol (1985) 2005;99(3):915–21.
22. Malikides N, Kessell A, Hodgson JL, et al. Bone marrow response to large volume blood collection in the horse. Res Vet Sci 1999;67(3):285–93.
23. Clark P, Mogg TD, Tvedten HW, et al. Artifactual changes in equine blood following storage, detected using the Advia 120 hematology analyzer. Vet Clin Pathol 2002;31(2):90–4.
24. Lilliehöök I, Tvedten H. Validation of the Sysmex XT-2000iV hematology system for dogs, cats, and horses. II. Differential leukocyte counts. Vet Clin Pathol 2009; 38(2):175–82.
25. Wise LN, Pelzel-McCluskey AM, Mealey RH, et al. Equine piroplasmosis. Vet Clin North Am Equine Pract 2014;30(3):677–93.
26. Johansson AM, Skidell J, Lilliehöök I, et al. Chronic granulocytic leukemia in a horse. J Vet Intern Med 2007;21(5):1126–9.
27. Kasashima Y, Ueno T, Tomita A, et al. Optimisation of bone marrow aspiration from the equine sternum for the safe recovery of mesenchymal stem cells. Equine Vet J 2011;43(3):288–94.
28. Bastos FZ, Barussi FCM, Santi TF, et al. Collection, processing and freezing of equine bone marrow cells. Cryobiology 2017;78:95–100.
29. Rowland AL, Navas de Solis C, Lepiz MA, et al. Bone marrow aspiration does not induce a measurable pain response compared to sham procedure. Front Vet Sci 2018;5:233.
30. Koch TG, Wen X, Bienzle D. Lymphoma, erythrocytosis, and tumor erythropoietin gene expression in a horse. J Vet Intern Med 2006;20(5):1251–5.
31. Morris DD, Whitlock RH. Relapsing idiopathic thrombocytopenia in a horse. Equine Vet J 1983;15(1):73–5.
32. Beeler-Marfisi J, Gallastegui Menoyo A, Beck A, et al. Gelatinous marrow transformation and hematopoietic atrophy in a miniature horse stallion. Vet Pathol 2011;48(2):451–5.
33. Miglio A, Pepe M, Felipe M, et al. Subleukaemic acute myeloid leukaemia with myelodysplasia in a horse. Equine Vet Educ 2019;31(6):e39–46.
34. Forbes G, Feary DJ, Savage CJ, et al. Acute myeloid leukaemia (M6B: pure acute erythroid leukaemia) in a thoroughbred foal. Aust Vet J 2011;89(7):269–72.
35. Boudreaux MK, Blue JT, Durham SK, et al. Intravascular leukostasis in a horse with myelomonocytic leukemia. Vet Pathol 1984;21(5):544–6.
36. Bienzle D, Hughson SL, Vernau W. Acute myelomonocytic leukemia in a horse. Can Vet J 1993;34(1):36–7.
37. Spier SJ, Madewell BR, Zinkl JG, et al. Acute myelomonocytic leukemia in a horse. J Am Vet Med Assoc 1986;188(8):861–3.
38. Blue J, Perdrizet J, Brown E. Pulmonary aspergillosis in a horse with myelomonocytic leukemia. J Am Vet Med Assoc 1987;190(12):1562–4.
39. Monteith CN, Cole D. Monocytic leukemia in a horse. Can Vet J 1995;36(12): 765–6.
40. Kelton DR, Holbrook TC, Gilliam LL, et al. Bone marrow necrosis and myelophthisis: manifestations of T-cell lymphoma in a horse. Vet Clin Pathol 2008;37(4): 403–8.

41. Coombs CC, Tallman MS, Levine RL. Molecular therapy for acute myeloid leukaemia. Nat Rev Clin Oncol 2016;13(5):305–18.
42. Meichner K, Kraszeski BH, Durrant JR, et al. Extreme lymphocytosis with myelomonocytic morphology in a horse with diffuse large B-cell lymphoma. Vet Clin Pathol 2017;46(1):64–71.
43. Badial PR, Tallmadge RL, Miller S, et al. Applied protein and molecular techniques for characterization of B cell neoplasms in horses. Clin Vaccine Immunol 2015;22(11):1133–45.
44. Cian F, Tyner G, Martini V, et al. Leukemic small cell lymphoma or chronic lymphocytic leukemia in a horse. Vet Clin Pathol 2013;42(3):301–6.
45. Long AE, Javsicas LH, Stokol T, et al. Rapid clinical progression of B-cell chronic lymphocytic leukemia in a horse. J Am Vet Med Assoc 2019;255(6):716–21.
46. Dascanio JJ, Zhang CH, Antczak DF, et al. Differentiation of chronic lymphocytic leukemia in the horse. A report of two cases. J Vet Intern Med 1992;6(4):225–9.
47. Bennett JM. Changes in the updated 2016: WHO classification of the myelodysplastic syndromes and related myeloid neoplasms. Clin Lymphoma Myeloma Leuk 2016;16(11):607–9.
48. Durando MM, Alleman AR, Harvey JW. Myelodysplastic syndrome in a quarter horse gelding. Equine Vet J 1994;26(1):83–5.
49. Pusterla N, Stacy BA, Vernau W, et al. Immunoglobulin A monoclonal gammopathy in two horses with multiple myeloma. Vet Rec 2004;155(1):19–23.
50. Eberhardt C, Malbon A, Riond B, et al. κ Light-chain monoclonal gammopathy and cast nephropathy in a horse with multiple myeloma. J Am Vet Med Assoc 2018;253(9):1177–83.

Coagulation Assessment in the Equine Patient

SallyAnne L. DeNotta, DVM, PhD[a], Marjory B. Brooks, DVM[b],*

KEYWORDS

- Hemostasis • Hemorrhage • Coagulopathy • Fibrinolysis
- Disseminated intravascular coagulation • Horse

KEY POINTS

- The coagulation cascade encompasses a series of cell membrane-associated reactions that culminate in the production of thrombin, which in turn transforms soluble plasma fibrinogen into an insoluble fibrin clot.
- Screening tests are broadly categorized as tests of primary hemostasis (platelet plug formation) or secondary hemostasis (fibrin clot formation).
- This article provides an overview of preliminary screening and definitive tests to assess equine platelet and coagulation pathways.
- This article reviews the hemostatic disorders most frequently encountered in clinical practice.

Although coagulopathies are relatively uncommon in equine patients, horses with clinical signs of hemorrhage and no apparent cause of vascular injury should be evaluated for underlying hemostatic defects. Systematically approaching such cases with the diagnostic algorithms provided in this article will enable clinicians to identify hemostatic defects in their patients early in the diagnostic workup.

HEMOSTASIS IN THE HORSE

The original cascade model of coagulation involves 2 distinct series of activation reactions (the intrinsic and extrinsic pathways) that converge to produce thrombin, which in turn transforms soluble plasma fibrinogen into an insoluble fibrin clot. Although this model is still useful for understanding in vitro coagulation, the refined cell-based model better reflects the in vivo formation of a hemostatic plug.[1] In this model, the availability and activation status of a variety of cell types regulate the localized formation of a platelet and fibrin plug. The cell-based model consists of 3 overlapping phases: initiation, amplification, and propagation (**Fig. 1**). The

[a] Large Animal Clinical Sciences, College of Veterinary Medicine, University of Florida, 2015 Southwest 16th Avenue, Gainesville, FL 32608, USA; [b] Comparative Coagulation Laboratory, Animal Health Diagnostic Center, Cornell University, Ithaca, NY 14850, USA
* Corresponding author. Comparative Coagulation Laboratory, Animal Health Diagnostic Center, Cornell University, 244 Farrier Road, Ithaca, NY 14853.
E-mail address: mbb9@cornell.edu

Vet Clin Equine 36 (2020) 53–71
https://doi.org/10.1016/j.cveq.2019.12.001
0749-0739/20/© 2019 Elsevier Inc. All rights reserved.

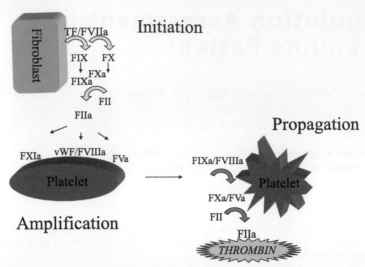

Fig. 1. Cell-based model of coagulation. Three phases of coagulation occur on different cell surfaces: (1) initiation on TF-bearing cells (eg, fibroblasts), (2) amplification on the platelet as it undergoes activation, and (3) propagation on the surface of activated platelets. In the initiation phase, the TF/factor VII complex (TF/coagulation factor VII) transforms factors IX and X to their active forms (FIXa and FXa, respectively), which generate trace amounts of thrombin (FIIa). In the amplification phase, thrombin mediates the activation of platelets and the coagulation cofactors (factors VIII and V). In the propagation phase, coagulation complexes (FIXa/FVIIIa and FXa/FVa) bind to activated platelet membranes and generate a large burst of thrombin that produces polymerized fibrin from fibrinogen.

initiation phase occurs on cells expressing tissue factor (TF), a membrane antigen constitutively expressed by most extravascular cells and inducibly expressed on some intravascular cells, particularly monocytes. TF exposed at sites of vascular injury participates in the formation of an active enzyme complex with coagulation factor VII to transform small amounts of the zymogen factors IX and X to their active forms: FIXa and FXa. If the procoagulant stimulus is sufficiently strong, the amplification phase follows initiation with reactions occurring primarily on the surface of platelets. Upon stimulation, platelets release procoagulant factors (eg, fibrinogen, factor V, and von Willebrand factor [vWF]) and provide a phospholipid surface for assembly of active coagulation complexes. In the propagation phase, the active coagulation factors combine with their cofactors to form the tenase (FIXa/FVIIIa) and prothrombinase (FXa/FVa) complexes, which interact to form FXa and thrombin (FIIa), respectively. This final phase results in a large-scale burst of thrombin sufficient to form an insoluble, cross-linked fibrin clot. Potent anticoagulant proteins, including TF pathway inhibitor, antithrombin (AT), and proteins C and S circulate in plasma and modulate each phase of hemostasis by neutralizing free active factors.[2]

As vascular defects heal, fibrinolytic pathways involving the plasma protease, plasmin, degrade cross-linked fibrin to reestablish blood flow. Plasmin is transformed from an inactive precursor, plasminogen, by tissue plasminogen activator and urokinase. This activation occurs most efficiently on the surface of mature fibrin. Free plasmin within the vascular space is neutralized by its inhibitor, antiplasmin, similar to the neutralization of free thrombin by AT. Plasmin degrades fibrin (or fibrinogen) to produce a series of progressive cleavage products. These fragments are referred to as fibrinogen/fibrin split products, or fibrinogen/fibrin degradation products (FDP). The terminal degradation fragments of fibrin are referred to as D-dimers.[3]

LABORATORY ASSESSMENT OF HEMOSTASIS

Coagulation screening tests are broadly categorized as tests of primary hemostasis (platelet plug formation) or secondary hemostasis (fibrin clot formation) (**Fig. 2**). Platelet plug formation involves a series of platelet activation steps (adhesion, aggregation, secretion) and requires vWF, an adhesive protein found in plasma, platelets, and the subendothelial matrix. Cross-linked fibrin is generated through the assembly of coagulation factor complexes that transform prothrombin to its active form, thrombin, which then acts on soluble fibrinogen to produce insoluble fibrin.

Sample Collection for Coagulation Assays

Appropriate sample collection and processing is critical for ensuring that assay results accurately reflect in vivo hemostatic conditions.[4] The key steps for sampling include atraumatic venipuncture and withdrawal of an exact volume of blood directly into tubes containing sodium citrate (3.2% or 3.8%) anticoagulant. Obtaining a complete draw directly into a blue top vacuum tube will provide the appropriate ratio of 1 part citrate to 9 parts blood. Blood may also be drawn directly from an indwelling intravenous catheter after withdrawal of a purge sample to remove any intraluminal heparin flush.[5] Blood drawn with no anticoagulant, into heparin (green top) or EDTA (purple top) anticoagulants, or into clot activator tubes, are not appropriate for coagulation screening assays. Plasma should be separated from cells, placed in a plastic or siliconized glass tube, and shipped chilled with an ice pack in an insulated container. Although statistically significant differences in clotting times have been reported for equine plasma stored frozen at −20°C versus fresh samples,[6] the noted changes were unlikely to be clinically relevant. A second study demonstrated stability of individual coagulation factor activities in equine plasma stored at −20°C for 90 days.[7]

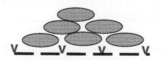

1⁰ Hemostasis Testing

Platelet aggregate formation

•Platelets & von Willebrand factor

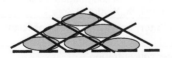

2⁰ Hemostasis Testing

Fibrin clot formation

•Coagulation factors & fibrinogen

Fig. 2. Schematic of Primary (1°) and secondary (2°) hemostasis. Primary hemostasis tests evaluate the components required for platelet plug formation (ie, functional platelets, vWF). Secondary hemostasis tests evaluate the interactions among coagulation factors that result in the generation of a cross-linked fibrin clot.

Coagulation kinetics vary among species, and coagulation laboratories should provide equine-specific reference ranges and controls whenever possible. If known laboratory values are not available, providing a normal control sample is recommended to aid in the interpretation of individual results.

Primary Hemostasis Tests

Several point-of-care (POC) tests and laboratory assays are available for assessing platelet quantity and function in horses (**Table 1**). Successful primary hemostasis

Table 1
Summary of hemostasis tests

Tests	Parameters Evaluated
Primary hemostasis (platelet and vWF)	
Platelet count and estimate from blood smear	Platelet number
TBT	Platelet adhesion, aggregation and vWF function
PFA 100 closure time[a]	Platelet adhesion, aggregation and vWF function
Platelet aggregometry[a]	Platelet aggregation in response to agonists (ie, ADP, collagen, PAF) Platelet dense granule secretion (ATP release)
Flow cytometry	Platelet membrane glycoproteins (ie, fibrinogen receptor complex) and activation markers (ie, bound fibrinogen, P-selectin, PS exposure, microparticle release)
vWF assays: vWF:Ag, vWF:CBA, vWF:RCo	vWF:Ag: Quantitative measure of vWF concentration vWF:CBA: vWF functional activity based on collagen binding vWF:Rco: vWF functional activity based on platelet agglutination
Secondary hemostasis (coagulation)	
ACT[a]	Coagulation factor activity (intrinsic and common pathway and fibrinogen)
Coagulation screening tests: APTT, PT, TCT, Fibrinogen	APTT: Activity of intrinsic and common pathway factors and fibrinogen PT: Activity of extrinsic and common pathway factors and fibrinogen TCT: Fibrinogen function Fibrinogen: Quantitative (and functional) fibrinogen
Coagulation factor assays	Specific activity of coagulation factors (factors II, V, VII, VIII, IX, X, XI, XII)
AT	AT inhibitory activity (inhibition of factor IIa or Xa)
D-dimer	D-dimer concentration
TEG/thromboelastometry[a]	Whole blood clot formation and fibrinolysis

Abbreviations: ADP, adenosine diphosphate; ATP, adenosine triphosphate; PAF, platelet activating factor; PFA, platelet function analyzer; PS, phosphatidylserine; PT, prothrombin time; TCT, thrombin clotting time; vWF:Ag, vWF antigen; vWF:CBA, vWF collagen binding activity; vWF:RCo, vWF ristocetin cofactor activity.
[a] Tests that must be performed at POC or within 1 hour of sample collection.

requires adequate platelet numbers as well as engagement of distinct cell surface receptors and a myriad of activation responses leading to platelet–surface attachment and formation of the platelet plug. Although quantitative deficiencies can be quickly ruled out with a simple platelet count, qualitative defects in platelet function or vWF should be suspected in horses with adequate platelet counts but clinical evidence of abnormal primary hemostasis, for example, mucosal hemorrhage, petechiae, ecchymoses.

Platelet count
Thrombocytopenia can occur as a primary or secondary condition in horses, and determination of platelet count should be performed as the initial screening test in horses with a suspected bleeding diathesis. Examination of a stained blood film is a rapid screen to assess platelet number (**Fig. 3**). Although the finding of at least 10 platelets per oil immersion field quickly rules out thrombocytopenia, a semiquantitative estimate of platelet count can be obtained by multiplying the average number of platelets per 10 oil immersion field × 15,000.

Note that spurious thrombocytopenia owing to platelet activation is very common in horses and examination of the feathered edge (and the body) of a smear (to detect platelet clumping) should be performed if instrument or manual counts indicate thrombocytopenia. Platelet activation can be minimized by careful venipuncture using an 18-gauge or larger needle and drawing blood slowly into a syringe preloaded with citrate anticoagulant (goal of approximately 9:1 blood-citrate ratio) and preparation of the smear as soon as possible after collection.

Template bleeding time
The template bleeding time (TBT) is an in vivo assay of platelet adhesion and aggregation, performed by making a superficial but defined length and depth wound, often in the forelimb, using a spring-loaded device.[8] Reported TBT for healthy horses ranges from 2 to 6 minutes and may be prolonged with both quantitative (thrombocytopenia) and qualitative (von Willebrand disease, Glanzmann thrombasthenia) disorders. Although simple to perform, the TBT is invasive with generally poor reproducibility and subject to interoperator variability and nonspecific prolongation.[9]

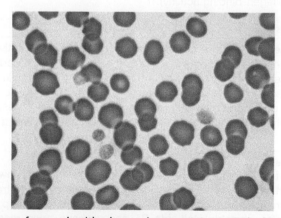

Fig. 3. Blood smear from a healthy horse demonstrates normal platelet numbers and morphologic features (stain: Wright's stain; original magnification ×400). (*Courtesy of* Dr. T. Stokol, Cornell University, Ithaca, NY.)

Platelet function analyzer

The platelet function analyzer (PFA-100 system, Siemens, Munich, Germany) is a table-top, POC instrument designed to measure in vitro platelet plug formation in human blood samples under conditions of high shear flow. The test end point (closure time) reflects the time for occlusion of a collagen/ADP-coated or collagen/epinephrine-coated aperture and the assay is used as a screening test for platelet adhesion and aggregation defects, including von Willebrand disease. It may also be useful for monitoring response to aspirin or clopidogrel therapy. Although this assay avoids some of the variability and patient discomfort of the TBT, it is influenced by some of the same nonspecific conditions, including low hematocrits and variations in blood viscosity. The PFA-100 has been evaluated in horses, with a reference range for the collagen/ADP closure time of 60 to 116 minutes.[10] The collagen/epinephrine assay, however, did not yield clinically useful results because closure times for some healthy horses using these cartridges exceeded the analyzer's cut-off value of 300 seconds.

Platelet aggregometry and flow cytometry

Platelet aggregation and secretion studies provide detailed and specific measures of platelet function. They require special instrumentation (aggregometers) and are performed by stimulating freshly isolated platelet-rich plasma samples with a panel of different agonist compounds. Flow cytometry also requires dedicated instrumentation and, for most studies, on-site blood collection for isolation of viable platelets. Cytometric assays evaluate platelet function via detection of membrane glycoproteins (including adhesion and aggregation receptors) and expression of specific activation markers, such as P-selectin, phosphatidylserine, and membrane-bound fibrinogen. The techniques are useful for characterizing hereditary platelet function defects (thrombopathias) and to study drug effects or disease pathogenesis.[11-17]

von Willebrand Factor

vWF is required for normal platelet adhesion and quantitative measurement is indicated in patients with prolonged TBT and/or PFA-100 closure times. In addition to quantitative measurement of vWF concentration (referred to as vWF antigen), vWF function can be evaluated based on a vWF-dependent platelet agglutination response (referred to as vWF ristocetin cofactor activity) or vWF's ability to bind immobilized collagen (vWF collagen-binding activity).[18]

Secondary Hemostasis Tests

Coagulation screening tests use specific reagents to sequentially activate distinct series of coagulation factors, or pathways, within the coagulation cascade (**Fig. 4**). Typically, the activated partial thromboplastin time (APTT), prothrombin time (PT), and fibrinogen are used together as screening tests to identify abnormalities in the intrinsic, extrinsic, and/or common coagulation pathways, and pattern of results from these tests can be helpful for identifying the specific defect in patients with abnormal hemostasis (**Fig. 5**).

Prothrombin time

This screening test evaluates the extrinsic and common pathways and their ability to convert fibrinogen to fibrin (see **Fig. 4**). This assay is traditionally performed in reference laboratories or with semiautomated benchtop coagulometric analyzers; however, portable stall-side PT assays have been recently evaluated and found to have good agreement and precision when compared with laboratory-based methods.[19] Different PT reagents and methods vary in their

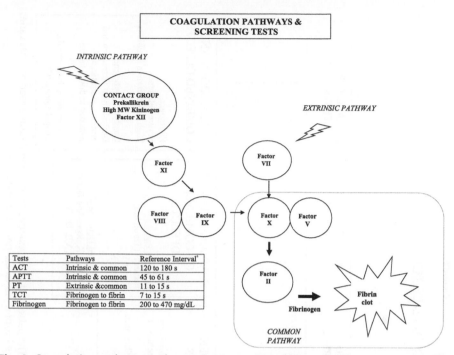

Fig. 4. Coagulation pathways and screening tests. Coagulation screening tests use specific reaction conditions to activate the intrinsic or extrinsic pathway. The activated partial thromboplastin time (APTT) and ACT initiate the intrinsic pathway through activation of the contact group factors (prekallikrein, high-molecular-weight kininogen, and factor XII). The prothrombin time (PT) test is configured with a TF reagent that initiates the extrinsic pathway through activation of factor VII. Thrombin generation results through activation of the common pathway factors (factors V, X, and II) to culminate in formation of a fibrin clot. The thrombin clotting time (TCT) and fibrinogen assays are measures of the final transformation of soluble fibrinogen to form the cross-linked fibrin clot. [a] Comparative Coagulation Laboratory, current 2019 values.

sensitivity to detect mild factor deficiencies; however, factor activities of less than 30% of normal should result in prolonged clotting times regardless of methodology. Prolonged PT indicate deficiencies of one or more of the following: factors V, VII, X, prothrombin (factor II), or fibrinogen.

Activated partial thromboplastin time

This screening test evaluates factors in the intrinsic and common pathways and their ability to convert fibrinogen to fibrin. The activated clotting time (ACT) is a simple POC test of this pathway, with expected ACT for horses of approximately 2 to 3 minutes. Unlike APTT, the ACT is more susceptible to nonspecific factors such as platelet count, platelet dysfunction, hematocrit, and plasma protease activity.[20] Prolonged APTT and/or ACT clotting times indicate deficiencies of one or more of the following: factors V, VIII, IX, X, XI, XII, prothrombin (factor II), or fibrinogen.

Note that severe hypofibrinogenemia (ie, <100 mg/dL) owing to hepatic synthetic failure or consumptive coagulopathies such as disseminated intravascular coagulation (DIC) may affect fibrin clot end point formation and result in prolongation of

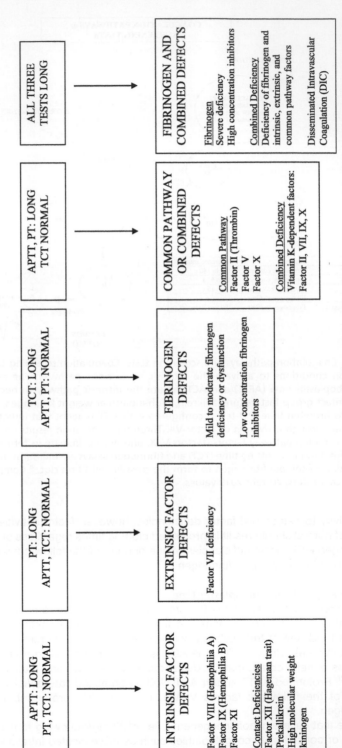

Diagnostic Algorithm for Coagulation Factor Deficiencies

COAGULATION SCREENING TESTS: APTT, PT, TCT

APTT: LONG
PT, TCT: NORMAL

INTRINSIC FACTOR DEFECTS

Factor VIII (Hemophilia A)
Factor IX (Hemophilia B)
Factor XI

Contact Deficiencies
Factor XII (Hageman trait)
Prekallikrein
High molecular weight kininogen

PT: LONG
APTT, TCT: NORMAL

EXTRINSIC FACTOR DEFECTS

Factor VII deficiency

TCT: LONG
APTT, PT: NORMAL

FIBRINOGEN DEFECTS

Mild to moderate fibrinogen deficiency or dysfunction

Low concentration fibrinogen inhibitors

APTT, PT: LONG
TCT NORMAL

COMMON PATHWAY OR COMBINED DEFECTS

Common Pathway
Factor II (Thrombin)
Factor V
Factor X

Combined Deficiency
Vitamin K-dependent factors:
Factor II, VII, IX, X

ALL THREE TESTS LONG

FIBRINOGEN AND COMBINED DEFECTS

Fibrinogen
Severe deficiency
High concentration inhibitors

Combined Deficiency
Deficiency of fibrinogen and intrinsic, extrinsic, and common pathway factors

Disseminated Intravascular Coagulation (DIC)

Fig. 5. Coagulation screening test algorithm for coagulation factor deficiencies. The pattern of abnormalities of the coagulation screening tests varies for different factor deficiencies. *Long:* prolongation of the patient's clotting time beyond 1.5 to 2.0 times the assay mean.

both the APTT and PT. Anticoagulant rodenticides that interfere with vitamin K recycling, for example, warfarin, brodifacoum, inhibit vitamin K-dependent factors (factors II, VII, IX, X) and result in prolongation of both the PT and APTT, but do not influence fibrinogen.

Thrombin clotting time
This qualitative fibrinogen test is performed by adding an excess of thrombin to the test plasma and measures the conversion of fibrinogen to fibrin. It is sensitive only to the deficiency, dysfunction, or inhibition of fibrinogen.

Coagulation factors
The specific procoagulant activity of individual coagulation factors and cofactors can be measured in modified APTT and PT screening tests configured with a series of single factor deficient plasmas.[21,22] Factor activities of the test samples are reported as a percentage or units per milliliter, compared with a standard plasma. In general, factor activities of greater than 50% are considered sufficient for normal hemostasis. The clinical relevance of factor activities of less than this value depends on the severity of the factor deficiency and whether only a single factor or multiple factors are involved.[23]

Coagulation inhibitors
AT and protein C are critical plasma inhibitors of coagulation. AT is a plasma serine protease inhibitor produced by the liver that inactivates factors IIa (thrombin) and Xa, thereby preventing active coagulation complex assembly and subsequent conversion of fibrinogen to fibrin. AT serves as the primary physiologic anticoagulant in circulation and deficiencies are associated with systemic hypercoagulability and thrombophilia.[23] Unfractionated and low-molecular-weight heparins act by markedly potentiating AT inhibitory activity. Protein C is a vitamin K-dependent protease that acts primarily at endothelial cell surfaces and with a cofactor, protein S, to degrade active factors VIII and V.[24] A lack of these physiologic inhibitors causes a relative hypercoagulable, prothrombotic state. Commercial chromogenic substrate assays can be adapted to measure equine AT and protein C activity and should include the use of same species standards and controls.[25]

Fibrinolysis Tests

Fibrin/Fibrinogen degradation products and D-dimer
Fibrin/Fibrinogen degradation products (FDP) are the end products of fibrinogenolysis or soluble fibrinolysis (cleavage of fibrinogen or non–cross-linked fibrin) or secondary lysis of cross-linked fibrin clots. D-dimer represent the terminal degradation product of fibrinolysis and consist of 2 cross-linked D domains of fibrin. Its presence is a specific indicator of plasmin's action on fibrin, rather than fibrinogen. In most assay systems, the plasma concentration of equine D-dimer is higher than human beings (and companion animals) with typical values for healthy horses ranging from 250 up to 1000 ng/mL.[26] Plasma concentrations of FDP and D-dimer are increased in response to any process that activates the coagulation cascade and results in clot formation and subsequent fibrinolysis. A nonspecific increase in FDPs may also be observed in response to increased fibrinogen levels. In horses, FDP and D-dimer have been found to be increased after colic surgery and in horses suffering from inflammatory gastrointestinal disease, and are one of the hallmarks of DIC.[27–29] High plasma D-dimer concentrations at admission were associated with nonsurvival in horses presented for colic and were found in horses with equine herpes virus-1 viremia,[30,31] a condition in

which microvascular thrombi form in several vascular beds, including the lungs, placenta, and spinal cord.

Viscoelastic methods: Thromboelastography and thromboelastometry

These POC assays record changes in the viscoelastic properties of whole blood from initiation of clot formation through fibrinolysis (**Fig. 6**).[32–34] Viscoelastic assays were developed as global tests of hemostasis and are able to characterize both hypocoagulable and hypercoagulable states. This method contrasts with traditional coagulation assays designed to evaluate isolated components of the coagulation cascade without the contribution of cellular elements. Specific activators such as TF or kaolin may be added to standardize reaction conditions and enhance the rate of coagulation. A modified hemoscopic thrombelastography (TEG) assay (PlateletMapping, Haemoscope) designed specifically to monitor response to antiplatelet drugs, performed poorly in an equine pharmacodynamic study of clopidogrel.[14] Erythrocytosis has been shown to induce hypocoagulabilty on TEG without concurrent changes in other coagulation parameters and is hypothesized to be a result of dilution of plasma coagulation factors by increased red blood cell mass.[35] Substantial variation has been documented in TEG reference intervals between differing laboratories, sample handling techniques, and between personnel within the same laboratory[36–38]; thus, this assay may be better suited for monitoring hemostatic trends over time in individual patients rather than making comparisons across individuals and institutions.

CLINICAL APPROACH TO HEMOSTATIC DEFECTS IN HORSES

The initial assessment of patients with signs of hemorrhage should aim to differentiate blood loss caused by vessel injury or vascular disease from a systemic failure of normal hemostasis. Large vessel (arterial/venous) defects typically present as acute blood loss from localized sites of vessel injury, whereas small vessel disorders or vasculopathies are more often associated with signs of bruising, edema, and systemic illness. Clinical signs suggestive of primary hemostatic defects (platelet and vWF disorders) include petechiae, ecchymoses, and mucosal hemorrhage (epistaxis, melena). Secondary hemostatic defects typically cause hematoma formation, hemarthrosis, and intracavitary bleeds. Severe bleeding diatheses often cause spontaneous hemorrhage, whereas mild to moderate forms may become apparent only after surgery or trauma. In the absence of a definitive diagnosis after simple POC screening tests, such as the platelet count and ACT, follow-up with submission of samples for coagulation profile and factor assays may be indicated (**Fig. 7**).

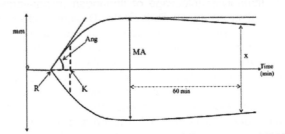

Fig. 6. Typical thromboelastogram with measured parameters: R = time to the initiation of clot formation, K = time for the tracing to achieve a set clot strength, Ang = Angle, the rate of clot formation, MA = maximum amplitude, the greatest clot strength, χ = clot strength at 60 minutes after MA, CL60 = 100 × (χ/MA). (*From* Epstein, KL et al. Thromboelastography in 26 healthy horses with and without activation by recombinant human tissue factor. J Vet Emerg Crit Care 2009:19(1): 96-101, 2009; with permission.)

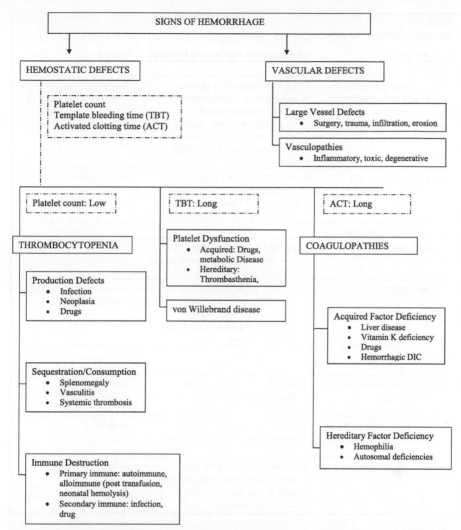

Fig. 7. Diagnostic algorithm for clinical signs of hemorrhage using POC tests. The findings of an abnormal platelet count, TBT, and activated coagulation time are indicators of hemostatic defects. DIC, disseminated intravascular coagulation.

Hereditary Hemostatic Disorders

Hereditary hemostatic defects are much less common than acquired disorders; however, hereditary platelet function defects, von Willebrand disease, and coagulation factor deficiencies have been identified in horses (**Table 2**). Hereditary defects are caused by mutations within genes coding for specific hemostatic proteins, resulting in impaired protein synthesis or production of dysfunctional proteins.

Platelet dysfunction

Hereditary platelet function defects, or thrombopathias, are broadly classified as abnormalities of platelet membrane receptors, signal transduction pathways, granule secretion, or membrane phospholipid flipping.[39] Glanzmann thrombasthenia refers

Table 2 Hereditary hemostatic defects		
Classification	Characteristic Laboratory Findings	Breeds
Platelet function defects		
Membrane glycoprotein defect (Glanzmann's thrombasthenia)	Long TBT, abnormal platelet adhesion and clot retraction; absent or diminished aggregation to all agonists, absent or reduced membrane fibrinogen receptor (αIIbβ3) complex	Thoroughbred, Quarter horse, Oldenburg
Undefined (reduced fibrinogen binding)	Long TBT, reduced platelet prothrombinase activity, diminished fibrinogen binding in response to thrombin	Thoroughbred
Von Willebrand disease		
Type 1 vWD	Long TBT, slight reduction FVIII:C, low vWF:Ag and proportionate reduction in vWF:RCo	Arabian
Type 2 vWD	Long TBT; slight reduction FVIII:C, low vWF:Ag with more pronounced reduction in vWF:Rco, decreased high MW vWF multimers	Thoroughbred, Quarter horse
Coagulation factor deficiencies		
Hemophilia A (factor VIII deficiency)	Long APTT, normal PT and fibrinogen, low FVIII:C	Thoroughbred, Standardbred, Quarter horse
Combined intrinsic factor deficiency (factors VIII, IX, XI)	Long APTT, normal PT and fibrinogen, low FVIII:C, FIX:C, FXI:C	Arabian
Prekallikrein deficiency	Long APTT, normal PT and fibrinogen, low prekallikrein activity, variable (or no) bleeding tendency	Belgian, Miniature horse

to quantitative and/or functional defects of the platelet membrane integrin, αIIbβ3. This complex (also termed glycoprotein IIbIIIa) acts as a fibrinogen receptor and plays a critical role in the formation of platelet aggregates in response to all agonists. Glanzmann thrombasthenia has been diagnosed in several breeds of horses, with 2 different mutations identified in the αIIb gene in Thoroughbreds and Quarter horses (see **Table 2**).[17,40–42] A platelet function defect, distinct from thrombasthenia, has also been reported in Thoroughbreds.[16] Affected horses demonstrated prolonged in vivo bleeding times, abnormal aggregation response to certain agonists, and impaired fibrinogen binding in a flow cytometric assay. The physiologic and molecular basis of this defect has yet to be discovered.

Von Willebrand disease
von Willebrand disease includes quantitative and functional defects of vWF. Three subtype classifications defined for human vWD are applicable to animals.[43] Type 1 vWD is a quantitative protein deficiency; patients have low vWF antigen with an equivalent reduction in vWF function (measured via agglutination or collagen binding). Type

2 vWD encompasses qualitative vWF defects; patients have moderate to severe vWF antigen deficiency with a disproportionate functional defect. Type 3 vWD is defined as the complete absence of vWF protein. Types 1 and 2 vWD have been identified in horses, with clinical signs of mucosal hemorrhage and prolonged postoperative hemorrhage (see **Table 2**).[44,45]

Coagulation factor deficiencies: Hemophilia

Hemophilias A and B are X-linked recessive traits caused by deficiency of coagulation factors VIII and IX, respectively. Both forms of hemophilia have been identified in horses and many other species; in all species hemophilia A is the more common form.[46–49] Typical of X-linked recessive traits, males that inherit a mutant factor VIII or IX gene express a bleeding tendency, whereas female carriers of a single mutant gene are clinically normal. Hemophilia is typically propagated by asymptomatic carrier females; on average, one-half the sons of a carrier are affected with hemophilia and one-half the daughters are carriers. Idiopathic, presumed autoimmune, acquired hemophilia A has also been described in a Thoroughbred mare treated successfully with immunosuppressants.[50] The clinical severity of hemophilia generally correlates with residual factor activity. Patients affected with severe hemophilia have residual factor activities of 1% or lower and experience frequent, spontaneous bleeds. Foals affected with severe hemophilia are often euthanized or die within a few days of birth owing to uncontrolled umbilical hemorrhage, hemarthrosis, blood loss anemia, or other manifestations of a bleeding diathesis. Even mild to moderate hemophilia carries a poor prognosis in horses compared with other species, owing to recurrent hemarthroses.

Coagulation factor deficiencies: Autosomal factor deficiencies

Deficiencies of the autosomal coagulation factors (fibrinogen and factors II, V, VII, X, XI, and XII) are less common than hemophilia and have not been well-characterized in horses. In human beings and dogs, most of these defects are recessive traits, with the severity of clinical signs generally related to residual factor activity. Factor XI deficiency, however, typically manifests as a bleeding tendency only after surgery or trauma and deficiency of contact factors (factor XII, prekallikrein) do not result in bleeding diathesis.[51,52] Coagulation factor deficiencies are detected by prolongation of coagulation screening tests, with definitive diagnosis based on results of specific factor activity assays (see **Table 2**).

Acquired Hemostatic Defects

In contrast with hereditary defects that typically affect only a single protein or pathway, acquired hemostatic defects are often complex, resulting from combined quantitative and functional defects of platelets and coagulation factors. Nevertheless, the diagnostic workup generally begins with standard basic POC tests (platelet count, ACT), the results of which are used to guide the selection of appropriate ancillary tests (see **Fig. 6**).

Thrombocytopenia

Normal equine platelet count ranges from approximately 100,000/μL to 250,000/μL. Spurious low platelet counts are common artifacts; therefore, the finding of thrombocytopenia should be confirmed by scanning a blood smear to detect any platelet clumping. Mild to moderate thrombocytopenia accompanies many disease processes and is a consistent finding in horses with *Anaplasma phagocytophilum* infection, piroplasmosis, and rattlesnake envenomation.[53–57] Abnormal bleeding attributable to thrombocytopenia rarely occurs at platelet counts of greater than 50,000/μL, with spontaneous hemorrhage most likely at platelet counts or less than 20,000/μL. Four general mechanisms cause thrombocytopenia: impaired platelet production, increased peripheral consumption, sequestration, and immune-mediated destruction. The diagnostic workup for thrombocytopenia aims to identify an underlying disease triggering one or more of these processes (**Table 3**). Production failure should be high on the differential diagnostic list for patients with thrombocytopenia combined with nonregenerative anemia and/or neutropenia (pancytopenia). Vasculitis and DIC shorten platelet lifespan and may result in clinically significant thrombocytopenia. Marked thrombocytopenia, with platelet counts of less than 20,000/μL, often develops in patients with immune-mediated platelet destruction. Primary immune-mediated thrombocytopenia implies an autoimmune disorder with production of antibodies directed against normal platelet antigens.[58] Secondary immune-mediated thrombocytopenia may develop in patients with infections, neoplastic disease, polyimmune syndromes, or after drug therapy.[58–60] Alloimmune thrombocytopenia is the clinical consequence of antiplatelet antibodies that develop after transfusion or during pregnancy.[61,62] In these cases, the transfusion recipient or pregnant mare recognizes platelet antigens unique to the donor blood product (or sire) and develops antibodies to the foreign immunogen. Neonatal thrombocytopenia develops after transfer of the alloantibodies to a nursing foal whose platelets express the antigen foreign to the mare.

Platelet dysfunction

Many common drugs and disease syndromes affect platelet function, including, but not limited to, liver failure, uremia, paraproteinemia, and DIC.[63–65] Drugs inhibit platelet activation and aggregation by a variety of different mechanisms. Aspirin and other nonsteroidal anti-inflammatory drugs act via inhibition of intraplatelet cyclo-oxygenase, resulting in impaired production of thromboxane and diminished platelet response to other agonists. Targeted antiplatelet agents' effects on equine platelet activation response have been described, including the fibrinogen receptor complex and ADP receptor blockade, and altered cyclic adenosine monophosphate metabolism.[12–14,66]

Table 3 Acquired hemostatic defects	
Classification	**Pathogenesis**
Thrombocytopenia	Decreased production (bone marrow disease: Infectious, neoplastic, aplastic) Increased utilization (vasculopathies, DIC, systemic thrombosis Sequestration (splenomegaly, acute endotoxemia) Increased destruction (primary or secondary immune-mediated, alloimmune)
Platelet dysfunction	Metabolic disease (uremia, hepatic failure, paraneoplastic hyperglobulinemia) Drugs (nonsteroidal anti-inflammatory agents, plasma expanders, sulfa drugs)
Coagulation factor deficiencies	Hepatic synthetic failure (acute hepatitis, necrosis, chronic cirrhosis) Vitamin K deficiency (cholestatic disease, vitamin K antagonist toxicities) DIC: Factor activation/secondary depletion (systemic inflammatory syndromes, gastrointestinal inflammation or strangulation, neoplasia, severe tissue injury)

Coagulopathies

Acquired coagulation factor deficiencies generally result from decreased factor synthesis, release of inactive factors, inhibition of factor activity, or excessive consumption and depletion of factors. Underlying disease conditions most often associated with coagulopathy include liver disease, vitamin K deficiency, drug or toxin exposure, and DIC (see **Table 3**).

The liver is the primary site of synthesis and clearance of most coagulation factors and their inhibitors. Liver failure (eg, secondary to hepatic necrosis, cirrhosis, acute hepatitis) sufficient to decrease hepatic synthetic capacity may result in coagulopathy owing to fibrinogen and factor deficiencies. Overt hemorrhage is an indicator of severe liver failure and a poor prognostic sign. In addition to synthetic failure, liver disease may impair hemostasis via vitamin K deficiency, dysfibrinogenemia, platelet dysfunction, and abnormal clearance of fibrinolytic activators, FDPs, and D-dimer.[67]

Vitamin K deficiencies result from inadequate intestinal absorption or impaired intrahepatic recycling. A constant source of vitamin K_1 is required for post-translational carboxylation of the vitamin K-dependent serine protease coagulation factors (factors II, VII, IX, and X). Warfarin (Coumadin), second-generation anticoagulant rodenticides (eg, Brodifacoum), and sweet clover contaminated with mold-producing dicoumarol all act to irreversibly block the activity of vitamin K epoxide reductase, a critical vitamin K processing enzyme. Anticoagulant rodenticide toxicity has been reported in horses, ponies, and miniature donkeys.[68,69] The combined deficiencies of factors II, VII, IX, and X causes prolongation of both the APTT and PT screening tests, however plasma fibrinogen concentrations are not affected.

Disseminated intravascular coagulation

DIC is an acquired hypercoagulable syndrome whose defining feature is the deposition of fibrin throughout the microvasculature.[70] The syndrome of DIC always develops secondary to an underlying disease and had been documented in horses with severe systemic inflammatory conditions and gastrointestinal disorders (**Fig. 8**).[71,72] The pathogenesis of DIC is complex; however, the DIC trigger secondary to inflammatory disease is believed to be the induced expression of TF in the vascular space. TF expression is upregulated on circulating monocytes and endothelial cells under the influence of inflammatory cytokines, thereby promoting activation of the coagulation cascade and the generation of thrombin. Regardless of inciting disease, the DIC process results in systemic, small vessel thrombosis. In a subset of patients, platelet and coagulation factor depletion ensue and culminate in a bleeding diathesis with overt hemorrhage.

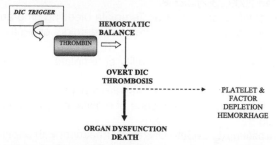

Fig. 8. Overview of DIC. A primary disease process perturbs regulation of hemostasis, resulting in systemic thrombin generation and formation of fibrin thrombi throughout the microvasculature. Thrombosis impairs organ function and may cause or contribute to mortality. In a subset of patients, hemorrhage develops secondary to depletion of platelets and coagulation factors.

The diagnosis of DIC is based on the presence of an initiating disease and a combination of clinical and laboratory abnormalities.[26,70] Hemorrhage is often subclinical, or absent in equine DIC, whereas hypercoagulability is common.[71] The classic laboratory features of DIC include low platelet count, prolonged APTT or PT, low fibrinogen concentration, low AT activity, and high FDP or D-dimer concentrations; however, a study of horses at necropsy revealed poor agreement between antemortem clotting profiles and histologic evidence of tissue fibrin deposition and DIC. These findings indicate that clinicians cannot rely solely on laboratory assays for the diagnosis of DIC.[72] Correction of the underlying disease process and targeted therapies based on clinical signs is the basis for successful management of DIC in horses. Anticoagulant therapy has not proven efficacious in human trials, but may be helpful for horses in the prothrombotic phases of DIC.[73] Blood and/or plasma transfusion is indicated for patients with severe thrombocytopenia or severe factor deficiencies and subsequent bleeding diathesis.

DISCLOSURE

The authors have nothing to disclose.

REFERENCES

1. Roberts HR, Hoffman M, Monroe DM. A cell-based model of thrombin generation. Semin Thromb Hemost 2006;32(Suppl 1):32–8.
2. Esmon CT. Coagulation inhibitors in inflammation. Biochem Soc Trans 2005; 33(Pt 2):401–5.
3. Medcalf RL. Fibrinolysis, inflammation, and regulation of the plasminogen activating system. J Thromb Haemost 2007;5(Suppl 1):132–42.
4. Meinkoth JH, Allison RW. Sample collection and handling: getting accurate results. Vet Clin North Am Small Anim Pract 2007;37(2):203–19.
5. Mackenzie CJ, McGowan CM, Pinchbeck G, et al. Comparison of two blood sampling techniques for determination of coagulation parameters in the horse: jugular venipuncture and indwelling intravenous catheter. Equine Vet J 2018;50(3):333–8.
6. Casella S, Giannetto C, Fazio F, et al. Assessment of prothrombin time, activated partial thromboplastin time, and fibrinogen concentration on equine plasma samples following different storage conditions. J Vet Diagn Invest 2009;21(5):674–8.
7. Wilson EM, Holcombe SJ, Lamar A, et al. Incidence of transfusion reactions and retention of procoagulant and anticoagulant factor activities in equine plasma. J Vet Intern Med 2009;23(2):323–8.
8. Kopp KJ, Moore JN, Byars TD, et al. Template bleeding time and thromboxane generation in the horse: effects of three non-steroidal anti-inflammatory drugs. Equine Vet J 1985;17(4):322–4.
9. Segura D, Monreal L. Poor reproducibility of template bleeding time in horses. J Vet Intern Med 2008;22(1):238–41.
10. Segura D, Monreal L, Espada Y, et al. Assessment of a platelet function analyser in horses: reference range and influence of a platelet aggregation inhibitor. Vet J 2005;170(1):108–12.
11. Brainard BM, Epstein KL, LoBato DN, et al. Treatment with aspirin or clopidogrel does not affect equine platelet expression of P selectin or platelet-neutrophil aggregates. Vet Immunol Immunopathol 2012;149(1–2):119–25.
12. Brainard BM, Epstein KL, LoBato DN, et al. Effects of clopidogrel and aspirin on platelet aggregation, thromboxane production, and serotonin secretion in horses. J Vet Intern Med 2011;25(1):116–22.

13. Hernandez D, Yeo WM, Brooks MB, et al. Effects of various antiplatelet drugs on ex vivo platelet activation induced by equine herpesvirus type 1. Am J Vet Res 2016;77(12):1366–73.
14. Brooks MB, Divers TJ, Watts AE, et al. Effects of clopidogrel on the platelet activation response in horses. Am J Vet Res 2013;74(9):1212–22.
15. Segura D, Monreal L, Perez-Pujol S, et al. Assessment of platelet function in horses: ultrastructure, flow cytometry, and perfusion techniques. J Vet Intern Med 2006;20(3):581–8.
16. Norris JW, Pratt SM, Auh JH, et al. Investigation of a novel, heritable bleeding diathesis of Thoroughbred horses and development of a screening assay. J Vet Intern Med 2006;20(6):1450–6.
17. Livesey L, Christopherson P, Hammond A, et al. Platelet dysfunction (Glanzmann's thrombasthenia) in horses. J Vet Intern Med 2005;19(6):917–9.
18. Rao ES, Ng CJ. Current approaches to diagnostic testing in von Willebrand Disease. Transfus Apher Sci 2018;57(4):463–5.
19. Berlin N, Kelmer E, Segev G, et al. Assessment of the CoaguChek-XS portable prothrombin time point-of-care analyzer for horses. J Vet Diagn Invest 2019; 31(3):448–52.
20. Rawlings CA, Byars TD, Van Noy MK, et al. Activated coagulation test in normal and heparinized ponies and horses. Am J Vet Res 1975;36(5):711–3.
21. Topper MJ, Prasse KW. Chromogenic assays for equine coagulation factors VII, VIII:C, IX, and X, and C1-esterase inhibitor. Am J Vet Res 1998;59(5):538–41.
22. Triplett DA, Smith MT. Routine testing in the coagulation laboratory. In: Triplett DA, editor. Laboratory evaluation of coagulation. IN: Chicago: American Society of Clinical Pathology Press; 1982. p. 27–52. Available at: https://www.ascp.org/content/learning/explore-books-and-journals.
23. Brooks MB. Coagulopathies and thrombosis. In: Ettinger SJ, Feldman BF, editors. Textbook of veterinary internal medicine. 5th edition. Philadelphia: W.B. Saunders, Co.; 2000. p. 1829–41.
24. Esmon CT. The protein C pathway. Chest 2003;124(3 Suppl):26S–32S.
25. Topper MJ, Prasse KW. Analysis of coagulation proteins as acute-phase reactants in horses with colic. Am J Vet Res 1998;59(5):542–5.
26. Stokol T, Erb HN, De Wilde L, et al. Evaluation of latex agglutination kits for detection of fibrin(ogen) degradation products and D-dimer in healthy horses and horses with severe colic. Vet Clin Pathol 2005;34(4):375–82.
27. Dallap BL. Coagulopathy in the equine critical care patient. Vet Clin North Am Equine Pract 2004;20:231–51.
28. Epstein KL. Coagulopathies in horses. Vet Clin North Am Equine Pract 2014;30: 437–52.
29. Cesarini C, Monreal L, Armengou L, et al. Progression of plasma D-dimer concentration and coagulopathies during hospitalization in horses with colic. J Vet Emerg Crit Care (San Antonio) 2014;24(6):672–80.
30. Cesarini C, Monreal L, Armengou L, et al. Association of admission plasma D-dimer concentration with diagnosis and outcome in horses with colic. J Vet Intern Med 2010;24(6):1490–7.
31. Goehring LS, Soboll Hussey G, Gomez Diez M, et al. Plasma D-dimer concentrations during experimental EHV-1 infection in horses. J Vet Intern Med 2013;27(6): 1535–42.
32. McMichael MA, Smith SA. Viscoelastic coagulation testing: technology, applications, and limitations. Vet Clin Pathol 2011;40(2):140–53.

33. Epstein KL, Brainard BM, Lopes MA, et al. Thromboelastography in 26 healthy horses with and without activation by recombinant human tissue factor. J Vet Emerg Crit Care (San Antonio) 2009;19(1):96–101.
34. Paltrinieri S, Meazza C, Giordano A, et al. Validation of thromboelastography in horses. Vet Clin Pathol 2008;37(3):277–85.
35. McMichael M, Smith SA, McConachie EL, et al. In-vitro hypocoagulability on whole blood thromboelastography associated with in-vivo expansion of red cell mass in an equine model. Blood Coagul Fibrinolysis 2011;22(5):424–30.
36. Jamieson CA, Hanzlicek AS, Payton ME, et al. Normal reference intervals and the effects of sample handling on dynamic viscoelastic coagulometry (Sonoclot) in healthy adult horses. J Vet Emerg Crit Care (San Antonio) 2018;28(1):39–44.
37. Thane K, Bedenice D, Pacheco A. Operator-based variability in equine thromboelastography. Am J Vet Res 2017;27(4):419–24.
38. Mendez-Andulo JL, Mudge MC, Vilar-Saavedra P, et al. Thromboelastography in healthy horses and horses with inflammatory gastrointestinal disorders an suspected coagulopathies. J Vet Emerg Crit Care (San Antonio) 2010;20(5):488–93.
39. Cattaneo M. Inherited platelet-based bleeding disorders. J Thromb Haemost 2003;1(7):1628–36.
40. Christopherson PW, van Santen VL, Livesey L, et al. A 10-base-pair deletion in the gene encoding platelet glycoprotein IIb associated with Glanzmann thrombasthenia in a horse. J Vet Intern Med 2007;21(1):196–8.
41. Macieira S, Rivard GE, Champagne J, et al. Glanzmann thrombasthenia in an Oldenbourg filly. Vet Clin Pathol 2007;36(2):204–8.
42. Sanz MG, Wills TB, Christopherson P, et al. Glanzmann thrombasthenia in a 17-year-old Peruvian Paso mare. Vet Clin Pathol 2011;40(1):48–51.
43. Brooks M. von Willebrand disease. In: Feldman BF, Zinkl JG, Jain NC, editors. Schalm's veterinary hematology. Philadelphia: Lippincott Williams Wilkins; 2000. p. 509–15.
44. Brooks M, Leith GS, Allen AK, et al. Bleeding disorder (von Willebrand disease) in a quarter horse. J Am Vet Med Assoc 1991;198(1):114–6.
45. Rathgeber RA, Brooks MB, Bain FT, et al. Clinical vignette. Von Willebrand disease in a Thoroughbred mare and foal. J Vet Intern Med 2001;15(1):63–6.
46. Norton EM, Wooldridge AA, Stewart AJ, et al. Abnormal coagulation factor VIII transcript in a Tennessee Walking Horse colt with hemophilia A. Vet Clin Pathol 2016;(45):96–102.
47. Littlewood JD, Bevan SA, Corke MJ. Haemophilia A (classic haemophilia, factor VIII deficiency) in a Thoroughbred colt foal. Equine Vet J 1991;23(1):70–2.
48. Henninger RW. Hemophilia A in two related quarter horse colts. J Am Vet Med Assoc 1988;193(1):91–4.
49. Mills JN, Bolton JR. Haemophilia A in a 3-year-old thoroughbred horse. Aust Vet J 1983;60(2):63–4.
50. Winfield LS, Brooks MB. Hemorrhage and blood loss-induced anemia associated with an acquired coagulation factor VIII inhibitor in a Thoroughbred mare. J Am Vet Med Assoc 2014;244:719–23.
51. Geor RJ, Jackson ML, Lewis KD, et al. Prekallikrein deficiency in a family of Belgian horses. J Am Vet Med Assoc 1990;197(6):741–5.
52. Turrentine MA, Sculley PW, Green EM, et al. Prekallikrein deficiency in a family of miniature horses. Am J Vet Res 1986;47(11):2464–7.
53. Zimmerman KL. Drug-induced thrombocytopenias. In: Feldman BF, Zinkl JG, Jain NC, editors. Schalm's veterinary hematology. Philadelphia: Lippincott Williams Wilkins; 2000. p. 472–7.

54. Sellon DC, Levine J, Millikin E, et al. Thrombocytopenia in horses: 35 cases (1989-1994). J Vet Intern Med 1996;10(3):127–32.
55. Davies RS, Madigan JE, Hodzic E, et al. Dexamethasone-induced cytokine changes associated with diminished disease severity in horses infected with Anaplasma phagocytophilum. Clin Vaccine Immunol 2011;18(11):1962–8.
56. Fielding CL, Pustural N, Magdesian KG, et al. Rattlesnake envenomation in horses: 58 cases (1992 – 2009). J Am Vet Med Assoc 2011;238(5):631–5.
57. Wise LN, Pelzel-McCluskey AM, Mealey RH, et al. Equine piroplasmosis. Vet Clin North Am Equine Pract 2014;30(3):677–93.
58. McGurrin MK, Arroyo LG, Bienzle D. Flow cytometric detection of platelet-bound antibody in three horses with immune-mediated thrombocytopenia. J Am Vet Med Assoc 2004;224(1):83–7, 53.
59. McGovern KF, Lascola KM, Davis E, et al. T-cell lymphoma with immune-mediated anemia and thrombocytopenia in a horse. J Vet Intern Med 2011;25(5):1181–5.
60. Cooper CJ, Keller SM, Arroyo LG, et al. Acute leukemia in horses. Vet Pathol 2018;55(1):15–172.
61. Buechner-Maxwell V, Scott MA, Godber L, et al. Neonatal alloimmune thrombocytopenia in a quarter horse foal. J Vet Intern Med 1997;11(5):304–8.
62. Ramirez S, Gaunt SD, McClure JJ, et al. Detection and effects on platelet function of anti-platelet antibody in mule foals with experimentally induced neonatal alloimmune thrombocytopenia. J Vet Intern Med 1999;13(6):534–9.
63. Segura D, Monreal L, Perez-Pujol S, et al. Effects of etamsylate on equine platelets: in vitro and in vivo studies. Vet J 2007;174(2):325–9.
64. Heidmann P, Tornquist SJ, Qu A, et al. Laboratory measures of hemostasis and fibrinolysis after intravenous administration of epsilon-aminocaproic acid in clinically normal horses and ponies. Am J Vet Res 2005;66(2):313–8.
65. Kingston JK, Bayly WM, Sellon DC, et al. Effects of sodium citrate, low molecular weight heparin, and prostaglandin E1 on aggregation, fibrinogen binding, and enumeration of equine platelets. Am J Vet Res 2001;62(4):547–54.
66. Rickards KJ, Andrews MJ, Waterworth TH, et al. Differential effects of phosphodiesterase inhibitors on platelet activating factor (PAF)- and adenosine diphosphate (ADP)-induced equine platelet aggregation. J Vet Pharmacol Ther 2003; 26(4):277–82.
67. Lisman T, Leebeek FW. Hemostatic alterations in liver disease: a review on pathophysiology, clinical consequences, and treatment. Dig Surg 2007;24(4):250–8.
68. Ayala I, Rodriguez MJ, Martos N, et al. Fatal brodifacoum poisoning in a pony. Can Vet J 2007;48(6):627–9.
69. McConnico RS, Copedge K, Bischoff KL. Brodifacoum toxicosis in two horses. J Am Vet Med Assoc 1997;211(7):882–6.
70. Kirby R, Rudloff E. Acquired coagulopathy VI: disseminated intravascular coagulation. In: Feldman BF, Zinkl JG, Jain NC, editors. Schalm's veterinary hematology, Vol. 5. Philadelphia: Lippincott, Williams & Williams; 2000. p. 581–7.
71. Dunkel B, Chan DL, Boston R, et al. Association between hypercoagulability and decreased survival in horses with ischemic or inflammatory gastrointestinal disease. J Vet Intern Med 2010;24(6):1467–74.
72. Cesarini C, Cotovio M, Rios J, et al. Association between necropsy evidence of disseminated intravascular coagulation and hemostatic variables before death in horses with colic. J Vet Intern Med 2016;30(1):269–75.
73. de Jonge E, van der Poll T, Kesecioglu J, et al. Anticoagulant factor concentrates in disseminated intravascular coagulation: rationale for use and clinical experience. Semin Thromb Hemost 2001;27(6):667–74.

Clinical Pathology in the Foal

Michelle Henry Barton, DVM, PhD, Kelsey A. Hart, DVM, PhD*

KEYWORDS

- Neonate • Foal • Hematology • Chemistry • Endocrinology

KEY POINTS

- There are important and significant differences in normal clinicopathologic test results between neonatal foals and mature horses.
- Failure to recognize these differences can lead to erroneous interpretation of neonatal clinical pathologic results.
- This article reviews common clinicopathologic test results in foals, relative to results reported for mature horses.

INTRODUCTION

The dynamic physiologic changes and unique diet during the neonatal period contribute to distinctive findings in clinical pathologic test results of healthy foals relative to healthy adult horses. When reporting results, most diagnostic laboratories provide reference intervals only for mature horses. Thus, failure to recognize the unique differences that occur in foals relative to adult horses can lead to erroneous interpretation of neonatal clinical pathologic results. Methodology also can profoundly affect the upper and lower limits reported for a reference interval, which can lead to erroneous interpretation when extrapolating results between laboratories. Ideally, reference intervals for healthy foals should be established within each diagnostic laboratory; however, funding limitations typically preclude provision of these data. Thus, this article reviews distinct features of common hematologic and serum biochemistry test results in foals, relative to mature horses. **Table 1** provides information on the clinicopathologic tests in foals that are different from adult horses.

Portions of this article were adapted from Barton MH. How to interpret common hematologic and serum biochemistry differences between neonatal foals and mature horses. American Association of Equine Practitioners Annual Convention, Las Vegas Proceedings 2015;61:125–129.
Department of Large Animal Medicine, University of Georgia College of Veterinary Medicine, Veterinary Medical Center, 2200 College Station Road, Athens, GA 30602, USA
* Corresponding author.
E-mail address: khart4@uga.edu

Table 1
Frequently observed differences in equine neonatal clinical pathologic tests results relative to adult horses

Result	Interpretation Relative to Adult Reference Intervals
Complete blood count	
Packed cell volume	Lower for first few months
Mean corpuscular volume and mean corpuscular hemoglobin concentration	Lower for first few months
White blood cells	Variable, but tend to be the same or slightly greater. Lymphopenia within first 1–3 d; physiologic lymphocytosis is not uncommon.
Coagulation	
Platelet count	Similar, although platelet function is reduced in the first 2 wk
Prothrombin and activated partial thromboplastin times	Same or longer for first 1–3 d
Fibrinogen concentration	Lower for first 1–3 d
Fibrin degradation product concentration	Greater for first 2 wk
Chemistry profile	
Total serum protein concentration	Lower for 4 to 6 wk
Serum globulin concentration	Lower for 4 to 6 wk
Blood or plasma lactate concentration	Single point measurements may be greater for at least 3 d
Creatinine concentration	May be greater for first 48 h, then drop below adult values while nursing vigorously
Urea nitrogen concentration	Initially the same at birth, but may drop below adult values during first few mo
Glucose concentration	Same or greater during first mo
Triglyceride concentration	Same or greater during first several mo
Total bilirubin and unconjugated bilirubin concentrations	Greater during the first 2 wk of life
Gamma glutamyltransferase activity	May be slightly greater for first 2 wk
Alkaline phosphatase activity	Greater during first year
Bile acid concentration	Greater during first 6 wk
Inorganic phosphate concentration	Greater during the first year
Creatine kinase activity	May be lower during the first year
Endocrine	
T_3 and T_4 concentrations	Greater than adults for first year
Cortisol concentrations	Initially greater at birth, then often falling below adult levels during the first several wk
Arterial oxygen tension	Lowest immediately after birth, then lower for first wk
Body fluids	
Cerebrospinal fluid protein and glucose concentrations	Greater for the first 2 mo

(continued on next page)

Table 1 (continued)	
Result	Interpretation Relative to Adult Reference Intervals
Peritoneal fluid total nucleated cell count and percentage of neutrophils	Lower for the first 2 mo
Urine	Specific gravity hypersthenuric at birth, then hyposthenuric; proteinuria for first 2 d: acidic
Bronchoalveolar lavage fluid	Higher percentage of macrophages and lower percentage of lymphocytes in the first mo

HEMATOLOGY
Erythrogram

Red blood cell (RBC) analytes are highly dynamic during the neonatal period. In general, immediately after birth, the RBC count, hemoglobin (Hgb) concentration, packed cell volume (PCV), and hematocrit (Hct) are similar to slightly higher than adult horses.[1-4] However, in most breeds, these values drop within 48 hours and continue to decrease to the low end or below the reference interval for mature horses.[5] For example, it is not unusual for the PCV/Hct to decrease in the first 48 hours of life from values of approximately 45% to 50% at birth to 35% to 40%, whereas absolute RBC counts do not decrease as dramatically.[1-4] The higher PCV at birth likely represents terminal placental transfer of blood and the physiologic stress of parturition inducing splenic contraction. The initial rapid reduction in PCV is due to a combination of adaptation to extrauterine life and hemodilution from blood volume expansion after ingestion of colostrum. The PCV, Hct, and Hgb continue to gradually decrease through the first month of life, most often with values falling in the low normal adult interval or even slightly below the lower limit of the adult interval.[1-4] The absolute RBC count often stays within adult intervals, thus the drop in Hct is mostly because neonatal erythrocytes become smaller (ie, microcytic) compared with adult RBCs and likely pack more densely. This is reflected in the mean corpuscular volume (MCV) values, which are similar to adult values at birth and then gradually decrease, reaching a nadir between 3 to 6 months that is below adult intervals.[5,6] The MCV in foals can remain lower than adults for up to a year.[5,6] Mean corpuscular hemoglobin concentration (MCHC) is derived by dividing the Hgb concentration by the Hct. In foals, the MCHC tends to be slightly lower to within normal limits, relative to adults.

Thus, collectively and compared with adults, foals often appear to be mildly anemic with smaller RBCs with less Hgb per cell. This "physiologic anemia" is common and appears to be due to a reduced stimulus for erythrogenesis and decreased iron availability.[2,7] Hypoxemia is a strong stimulus for erythropoiesis. After birth, foal RBCs have higher amounts of 2,3-diphosphoglycerate than adult RBCs, a feature that is typical of immature RBCs.[7] The 2,3-diphosphoglycerate facilitates the release of oxygen in tissues; thus, greater concentrations in the neonate may curtail erythrogenesis. Iron and ferritin concentrations drop rapidly in the first few days, and total iron binding capacity is higher in the neonatal foal than the adult; this may be in part because of the low iron content of milk versus colostrum and depletion of fetal iron stores.[5,7] Serum ferritin concentrations in foals increase with age and reach values consistent with adult horses by approximately 9 months of age.[8] The concurrent presence of microcytes is supportive evidence for functional iron deficiency.[6] Relative lack of iron availability and the associated physiologic anemia rarely result in clinical abnormalities in the neonatal period. However, it would be atypical for the PCV to drop below 20% in a foal or to decrease rapidly, in which case additional diagnostic tests would be warranted. Iron deficiency anemia was described in a hospitalized neonatal foal with concurrent sepsis, and was associated with low milk iron concentrations in the dam.[9]

It should be noted that breed differences have been noted particularly in RBC indices in horses. Physiologic anemia and the changes in RBC indices seen in foals may be less dramatic in draft breeds, as compared with light-breed horses.[3] In one study, the degree of anemia in Arabian foals during the first year of life was more pronounced than in thoroughbred or quarter horse foals.[10] Donkey foals follow the same trend as light-breed foals.[4,11] However, it is important to note that these studies were conducted in different laboratories and direct comparison of specific test results is difficult.

Leukogram

Total leukocyte and absolute neutrophil counts tend to be the same or slightly exceed adult values, whereas lymphocyte counts tend to be the same or below mature horse reference intervals during the first day after birth.[6] Total leukocyte and mature neutrophil counts usually remain comparable to or slightly higher than adult levels during the first year of life.[6] Band neutrophils are expected to remain low (usually <250/µL) during the neonatal period. During the first few days, absolute lymphocyte counts may fall below 1000/µL. The higher neutrophil-to-lymphocyte ratio may be in part because of the endogenous release of cortisol at parturition. The lack of the parturition cortisol surge in otherwise "healthy" premature foals is typically accompanied by a characteristic neutropenia at birth, wherein the severity of the neutropenia correlates with the likelihood of survival.[12] Lymphocyte counts are lowest at birth, and increase steadily during the first year of life to reach adult levels by 3 to 12 months of age.[6] However, physiologic lymphocytosis subsequent to catecholamine release can result in a rapid increase in the total lymphocyte count during periods of stress or illness. Circulating eosinophils are typically not seen in a standard 100-cell differential leukocyte count in foals.

COAGULATION

Coagulopathy is common in critically ill neonates, with one recent study reporting at least 1 abnormal coagulation test result in 64% of foals with septic shock.[13] Comprehensive assessment of hemostasis can include determining the platelet count, prothrombin (PT) and activated partial thromboplastin times (aPTT), fibrinogen concentration, fibrin degradation products (FDP), or D-dimer concentration, and perhaps antithrombin (AT) activity. As for many clinical pathologic tests, methodology can directly impact the reference interval, and this is particularly true for coagulation testing. Platelet counts are most accurate if the blood is collected into sodium citrate as the anticoagulant.[14–16] Platelet counts are the same or slightly higher in foals during the first few days of life, and then become comparable to adult values.[17–19] Despite comparable platelet numbers, platelet function is impaired in the first week of life, being less responsive to factors that initiate aggregation.[19] The PT and aPTT are the same or longer, and fibrinogen concentrations are lower in the foal's first few days of life when compared with the adult horse.[13,17–19] Concentrations of FDPs are significantly higher in foals than adult horses for at least 2 weeks.[17,18] Antithrombin activity is significantly lower during the first month of life, with mean activity approximately one-half adult values at birth.[17,18] D-dimer concentrations are lowest at birth in the foal, and increase during the first week to month of life,[20] but were not different between foals 1 to 6 months of age and adult horses.[21] Studies directly comparing D-dimer concentrations between healthy neonatal foals and adult horses are not currently available.

BIOCHEMISTRY
Proteins

The total protein concentration varies considerably in the first 24 to 36 hours, depending on the timing of absorption of colostral immunoglobulin. Presuckle total protein concentration is usually less than 5 g/dL and thus would fall below adult reference intervals. Post-suckle total protein concentrations usually are greater than 6 g/dL, but may remain in the low to slightly below adult reference intervals for several weeks. Albumin concentrations tend to stay within adult reference intervals; thus, the albumin-to-globulin ratio is usually normal or slightly lower than adult horses.[22] Although total protein concentration is not a reliable indicator of transfer of passive immunity, a low albumin-to-globulin ratio may be supportive evidence for partial or complete failure of passive transfer[22] and should be verified by a more specific test quantifying immunoglobulin G concentrations.

Serum Amyloid A

Although nonspecific as to the disease, increased plasma concentration of the acute phase protein serum amyloid A (SAA) correlates well with the presence of systemic inflammatory and infectious disease. Healthy foals younger than 3 days old have a range of SAA concentrations (0–27.1 mg/L, 95% confidence interval) within that reported for healthy adult horses.[23] The mean concentration in this study was greatest in foals at 2 days of age.

Electrolytes

The only subtle difference in sodium concentration in foals relative to adult horses is that the sodium concentration may be at the low end of adult reference intervals in the first 24 to 48 hours. This is most likely due to mild hemodilution following osmotic fluid expansion after absorption of colostral immunoglobulins. Otherwise, sodium, potassium, chloride, bicarbonate, and magnesium concentrations typically remain stable during the neonatal period with no significant differences relative to the mature adult horse.[24] It should be noted that the classic electrolyte changes anticipated with uroperitoneum (hyperkalemia, hyponatremia, hypochloremia, hypocalcemia) will be less apparent in foals that are concurrently receiving intravenous fluid therapy.[25,26] Inorganic phosphate concentrations are similar to adult values at birth, and then gradually increase over the first 2 months and may be slightly higher than adult values during the first year of life because of rapid bone growth.[22] For example, adult phosphate concentrations usually are less than 4 mg/dL, whereas foal phosphate concentrations can range between 6 and 8 mg/dL in the first year of life. At birth, total and ionized calcium concentrations are 25% to 30% higher than adult reference intervals, but decrease rapidly to 20% lower than adult values in the first few hours.[27] Total and ionized calcium concentrations stabilize in the first few days of life and then remain within adult reference intervals.

Lactate

Hyperlactatemia is associated with tissue hypoxia or reduced perfusion, but also can occur with increased metabolic demand, as would occur with sepsis, shivering, or seizures.[27] Reported blood or plasma lactate concentrations measured at or shortly after birth have been reported to be as high as 4.9 ± 1.0 mmol/L in healthy foals and may remain higher than adult values for at least 3 days.[28] The reason for this relative increase in lactate concentration in apparently healthy foals is unknown. Serial monitoring of blood lactate concentration may be more helpful than single point measurement in the first few days of life, as concentrations decrease with age.[29] Blood lactate concentrations in foals between 1 and 6 months old are the same as concentrations in adults.[28]

Kidney

Creatinine concentrations are often higher (2.5 ± 0.6 mg/dL) than adult values in the first 24 to 36 hours of life.[22] In a retrospective study on hypercreatinemia in foals younger than 2 days old, the term "spurious" hypercreatinemia was used to describe azotemia in a group of neonatal foals that had increased creatinine concentrations at admission (13.6 ± 7.5 mg/dL) without concurrent evidence of renal dysfunction.[30] Spurious hypercreatinemia is commonly reported in foals with neonatal encephalopathy and maternal placental insufficiency.[30–32] However, foals with spurious hypercreatinemia without renal disease typically have normal urea nitrogen concentrations and the creatinine concentration usually steadily decreases to within reference intervals within the first 72 hours of life.[30] Endogenous creatinine is removed from the fetal circulation via the placental circulation. Thus, higher creatinine concentrations in the first day of life more likely reflect placental dysfunction rather than primary renal disease. Creatinine concentrations frequently fall below 1.0 mg/dL in the well-hydrated and vigorously nursing foal. Urea nitrogen values are similar to adult values at birth and then tend to drop below the lowest limit of adult reference intervals (approximately 12 mg/dL) from the first few days of life to 5 months of age.[22]

Liver

The liver serves many diverse roles in normal homeostasis, including protein, lipid, and carbohydrate metabolism; vitamin storage; hemostasis; detoxification; and excretion. The total bilirubin concentration, primarily consisting of unconjugated or indirect bilirubin, is significantly higher in neonatal foals than mature horses, peaking in the first week (up to 5 mg/dL) and remaining high during the first 2 weeks of life.[22,33,34] Unconjugated bilirubin concentrations are often 2 to 4 times the adult mean value during this time and are higher in premature foals than foals of appropriate gestational age.[32] Physiologic unconjugated hyperbilirubinemia of human neonates is caused by the shorter RBC life span, reduced hepatocellular uptake of bilirubin, reduced activity of UDP-glucuronosyltransferase, the enzyme responsible for conjugation, and increased intestinal uptake of bilirubin by a factor, which has not yet been identified, in breast milk.[35] Physiologic hyperbilirubinemia in neonates can be further exacerbated by anorexia. Physiologic hyperbilirubinemia, coupled with physiologic anemia during this period (see erythrogram above), can be misconstrued as evidence of hemolytic anemia. Bilirubin concentrations in donkey foals tend not to be as high as horse foals, and often are within adult donkey reference intervals.[11,36]

Foals have less stored hepatic glycogen than adult horses, and are not yet hindgut fermenters. Thus, plasma glucose concentrations in foals tend to be highly variable, depending on demand, stress, and nursing frequency. In general, glucose concentrations are usually higher than adult values during the first month of life, often exceeding twice adult upper reference limits. Likewise, triglyceride concentrations are highly variable and reflective of nursing. Triglyceride concentrations may be as high as 340 mg/dL in healthy foals in the first few months of life, whereas adult values rarely exceed 50 mg/dL.[22,33,34]

In general, liver-associated enzymes are higher in neonatal foals and have more variability between individuals, as compared with adults.[33,37] The activities of the liver-specific enzymes, sorbitol dehydrogenase (SDH) and gamma glutamyltransferase (GGT), are either similar to adult values or slightly increased in the first 2 weeks, and then increase between 1 and 4 weeks of life.[33,34,37] Unlike ruminant neonates, there is little GGT in colostrum, and thus GGT activities do not correlate with transfer of passive immunity in foals. Gamma glutamyltransferase activity is significantly increased in premature foals.[32] In a retrospective case-control study on 147 foals younger than 30 days old with increased SDH or GGT activities, foals with higher liver enzyme activities were more likely to be septic, and septic foals were less likely to survive than were foals without sepsis. However, high liver enzyme activities alone were not a useful negative prognostic indicator.[38] Alkaline phosphatase (ALP) activity is very high in the first week of life (up to 3000 U/L) and may remain above the upper reference limit for adult horses for the first year of life.[22,34,39] The relatively higher ALP activity of neonatal foals is primarily due to the bone isoenzyme[39] and increased release associated with osteoblastic activity during rapid bone growth.

Although foals consume an exclusive milk diet, the colonic microbiota produce less ammonia as a by-product of protein catabolism. Thus, plasma ammonia concentrations are lower in the neonatal period, which may skew its accuracy as an indicator of hepatic function.[27] Bile acid concentrations are also frequently used as a functional assay of the liver,[33] but are significantly higher than mean adult values during the first 6 weeks of life, with radioimmunoassay values exceeding enzymatically determined values.[33] Increased bile acid concentration in the neonatal period may be due to upregulation of hepatic production, reduced excretion into the bile, unique effects of intestinal flora on the bile acid composition of the neonate, or enhanced intestinal absorption or uptake from the portal circulation.

Collectively, misinterpretation of higher bilirubin and bile acid concentrations and higher GGT, SDH, and ALP activities could erroneously lead to a diagnosis of liver disease in the neonatal period.

Muscle

Aspartate aminotransferase (AST) activity is primarily associated with muscle, although some AST activity is also found in the liver. In foals, AST activity tends to be the same or slightly lower than adult values during the first week of life, but values tend to remain within adult reference intervals as they continue to exercise and grow.[22,37] Increased AST activity has been reported in premature foals.[32] Creatine kinase (CK) activity is fairly comparable to adult intervals, although some individual foal's values may dip below adult values in the first few months.[22] Increased CK activity is reported in 62% of foals with neonatal encephalopathy[31] and is likely the result of placentitis, perinatal asphyxia, trauma at birth, prolonged recumbency, and seizures that often accompany neonatal encephalopathy.[27]

Endocrine

As would be expected for an endocrine axis that plays a key role in growth and development and metabolism, the thyroid axis is upregulated in the foal. During the first month of life, thyroid hormone concentrations are increased and can reach levels 10 to 14 times higher than those seen in healthy adult horses.[40,41] Total triiodothyronine (T3) and total thyroxine (T4) concentrations increase further after birth, peaking at 2 to 3 days of age, then decrease to reach adult levels by approximately 1 month of age.[40–43] Free T3 and free T4 concentrations are also increased at birth, but return to adult levels by 2 weeks of age.[40] Thyrotropin-stimulating hormone concentration is high at birth but decreases to adult levels by 12 hours of age.[40] Thyroid dysfunction is more common and may have more substantial consequences in neonatal foals than in adult horses. Nonthyroidal illness syndrome (previously known as "euthyroid sick syndrome"), characterized by decreased total and free T3 and T4 concentrations and increased reverse T3 concentrations, has recently been described in critically ill neonatal foals, and appears to be associated with a poorer prognosis.[40,44,45] There does appear, however, to be some overlap in thyroid hormone concentrations between healthy and sick foals, so at present, specific cutoff values for diagnosis of nonthyroidal illness syndrome in neonatal foals have not been proposed.

A fetal cortisol surge is a critical physiologic event at parturition in both the mare and foal. Adrenocorticotropic hormone (ACTH) concentrations are greatest at birth (up to ∼1000 pg/mL),[46,47] but rapidly decrease to levels consistent with approximate adult values within 48 hours. Likewise, cortisol concentrations are also highest in the first 30 minutes after birth (6–13 μg/dL), but drop within 48 hours, often falling below mean adult horse values during the first few weeks of life.[46,47] Premature foals have significantly higher ACTH and lower cortisol (often <1 μg/dL) concentrations at birth than full-term foals, due to late maturation of the hypothalamic-pituitary-adrenal axis in the neonatal foal.[12] Newborn foals also exhibit impaired responses to exogenous ACTH, as evidenced by ACTH stimulation tests. Insulin-induced cortisol responses in foals within 12 hours of birth are less than half of the responses achieved in 7-day-old to 14-day-old foals,[48] and healthy term neonatal foals aged 1 to 7 days are reported to have approximately half the magnitude of cortisol response to ACTH stimulation testing than adult horses.[46,49] This decreased adrenocortical responsiveness appears to persist during the first few months of life, as 12-week-old foals show significantly greater cortisol responses to a low-dose (0.1 μg/kg) ACTH stimulation test than younger foals.[50]

Despite decreased total cortisol concentrations compared with adult horses in the neonatal period after the peri-partum surge, neonatal foals have markedly decreased availability of the primary cortisol-binding protein, cortisol-binding globulin, which results in significantly higher circulating free, biologically active, cortisol in neonatal foals (30%–60% free) compared with adult horses (5%–10% free) during the first few weeks of life.[51] This increased availability of free cortisol likely offsets the limited cortisol synthetic capacity during the same time period in newborn foals, but does result in more rapid cortisol clearance in foals,[52] which could predispose foals to cortisol insufficiency during periods of intense or prolonged stress, such as severe illness.

Recently, other corticosteroids produced in the adrenal glands and the central nervous system have been demonstrated to play a key role in fetal and neonatal central nervous system function in the foal, suggesting a potential role for altered concentrations of these so-called neurosteroids in the etiology of equine neonatal encephalopathy.[53] Measurement of some of these compounds, such as allopregnanolone, may prove to have diagnostic or prognostic utility in ill or suspect foals with neonatal encephalopathy, but quantification of these neurosteroids is not commercially available to date.[54]

ARTERIAL BLOOD GAS ANALYSIS

Typically, in the mature horse, the expected arterial oxygen tension (P_aO_2) range is 90.2 ± 2.2 to 101.7 ± 1.6 mm Hg, with values less than 80 mm Hg indicative of hypoxemia.[55] As one would expect, inflation of the lungs and closing of shunts used in fetal circulation result in rapid changes in arterial blood gas analysis post parturition. Relative to a sample taken from a standing foal, it is important to note that P_aO_2 can be significantly decreased by up to 14 mm Hg when the sample is taken with the foal in lateral recumbency.[27] Foals are hypoxemic immediately after birth, with normal P_aO_2 as low as 40 to 50 mm Hg while in lateral recumbency. Arterial oxygen tension obtained from foals in lateral recumbency often remains ≤80 mm Hg for the first 24 hours of life, but values approach the lower limit of adult reference intervals between 1 and 3 days of life.[56] The arterial carbon dioxide tension (P_aCO_2) is only slightly higher than the expected adult mean in the first 24 hours and then falls within expected adult interval of 40 to 44 mm Hg.[56]

BODY FLUID ANALYSES
Cerebrospinal Fluid

Compared with healthy adult horses, the total nucleated cell count (≤5 cells/μL) and differential cell count (predominately mononuclear cells) in cerebrospinal fluid (CSF) are the same in neonatal foals. Increased CSF protein concentration is associated with various disorders, including meningitis, hemorrhage, vasculitis, or trauma. Reduced glucose concentrations in the CSF of foals reflect either hypoglycemia (CSF glucose is approximately 80% of the plasma glucose value) or septic meningitis.[57] However, it is important to note that the total protein and glucose concentrations of CSF in foals younger than 2 days old (109.0 ± 9.7 mg/dL and 98.8 ± 12.0 mg/dL, respectively) are essentially twice the values reported in adult horses.[58] Total protein and glucose concentrations in CSF gradually decrease in healthy foals to approach adult values by 2 months of age.[58]

Synovial Fluid

The interpretation of synovial fluid analysis for foals is essentially the same as for adult horses. The nucleated cell count is usually low (≤300 cells/μL) and the protein concentration is less than 2 g/dL.[27]

Peritoneal Fluid

In general, abdominocentesis is not performed in the neonate as routinely as in the adult horse. Nonetheless, the mean total nucleated cell count in peritoneal fluid in foals younger than 2 months old is reportedly lower (1418 ± 1077 cells/μL) than most reported values for adult horses.[59] The percentage of neutrophils (15%) is also lower than what is reported for adults. Peritoneal fluid protein concentrations are lower than adult horses; however, when measuring peritoneal fluid protein concentration in foals with a refractometer, concentrations are below the detection limit (2.5 g/dL) and are indistinguishable from healthy adult values.[59]

Urine

The urine specific gravity (USG) of the first voided urine is typically hypersthenuric (USG >1.030), but by 2 days of life, urine should become and remain hyposthenuric (USG <1.008) in nursing foals with normal renal function. As foals consume less milk with age, and the medullary concentration gradient matures, USG becomes more variable. With the excretion of microglobulins associated with ingestion and absorption of colostral immunoglobulins, proteinuria (up to +2) is normal in the first 2 to 3 days of life. Small numbers of leukocytes and RBCs may be normally present in the urine for first 2 days of life and are likely from post-foaling umbilical cord rupture before complete closure of the urachus.[27] Foal urine is more acidic (pH 5.5–8.0) relative to the adult horse. Urine GGT-to–urine creatinine ratios can be used to investigate renal tubular damage in foals and is within the reference range of healthy adult horses (8.16 ± 5.7).[60]

Bronchoalveolar Lavage

Differences in the percentages of nucleated cells normally found in bronchoalveolar lavage fluid (BALF) have been reported.[61] Foals have a higher proportion of macrophages in BALF with the highest proportion of macrophages occurring at 1 month of age (median: 87.3%), differing significantly from adults (median: 48.7%). The proportion of lymphocytes in the BALF was considerably lower in neonatal foals younger than 1 month old (median: <5%), compared with adults (median: 45.8%). The neutrophil percentage was highest in foals aged 1 week (13.7%) but not significantly different from adult horses.

SUMMARY

There are many dynamic changes that occur in clinicopathologic values during the neonatal period. Some of these are the result of transition from the unique intrauterine environment to life after parturition and some are the simply because additional time is needed for maturation. Without having a reference interval for foals, interpretation of clinicopathologic data in the neonatal period must be done vigilantly. Because most diagnostic laboratories only report adult reference intervals, familiarity with the most common differences relative to adult horses will help reduce interpretation error during the neonatal period.

REFERENCES

1. Harvey JW, Asquith RL, McNulty PK, et al. Haematology of foals up to one year old. Equine Vet J 1984;16:347–53.
2. Harvey J. Normal hematologic values. In: Koterba A, Drummond W, Kosch P, editors. Equine clinical neonatology. Philadelphia: Lea and Febiger; 1990. p. 561–70.
3. Aoki T, Ishii M. Hematological and biochemical profiles in peripartum mares and neonatal foals (heavy draft horse). J Equine Vet Sci 2012;32:170–6.
4. Sgorbini M, Bonelli F, Rota A, et al. Hematology and clinical chemistry in Amiata donkey foals from birth to 2 months of age. J Equine Vet Sci 2013;33:35–9.
5. Harvey JW, Asquith RL, Sussman WA, et al. Serum ferritin, serum iron, and erythrocyte values in foals. Am J Vet Res 1987;48:1348–52.
6. Faramarzi B, Rich L. Haematological profile in foals during the first year of life. Vet Rec 2019;184:503.
7. Kohn CW, Jacobs RM, Knight D, et al. Microcytosis, hypoferremia, hypoferritemia, and hypertransferrinemia in standardbred foals from birth to 4 months of age. Am J Vet Res 1990;51:1198–205.
8. Ohya T, Kondo T, Yoshikawa Y, et al. Change of ferritin-binding activity in the serum of foal after birth. J Equine Sci 2011;22:73–6.
9. Fleming KA, Latimer KS, Barton MH. Iron deficiency anemia in a neonatal foal. J Vet Intern Med 2006;20:1495–8.
10. Moruzzi MM, Orozco CAG, Martins CB, et al. Haematological parameters in Arabian foals./Estudo de parâmetros hematológicos de potros da raça puro sangue Árabe. Ars Vet 2007;23:129–33.
11. Veronesi MC, Gloria A, Panzani S, et al. Blood analysis in newborn donkeys: hematology, biochemistry, and blood gases analysis. Theriogenology 2014;82:294–303.
12. Silver M, Knox J, Cash RSG, et al. Studies on equine prematurity. 2. Post natal adrenocortical activity in relation to plasma adrenocorticotrophic hormone and catecholamine levels in term and premature foals. Equine Vet J 1984;16:278–86.

13. Bentz AI, Wilkins PA, Boston RC, et al. Prospective evaluation of coagulation in critically Ill neonatal foals. J Vet Intern Med 2009;23:161–7.

14. Ehrmann C. An overview of equine hematology. Prakt Tierarzt 2015;96:480–8.

15. Hinchcliff KW, Kociba GJ, Mitten LA. Diagnosis of EDTA-dependent pseudo-thrombocytopenia in a horse. J Am Vet Med Assoc 1993;203:1715–6.

16. Williams TL, Archer J. Effect of prewarming EDTA blood samples to 37 degrees C on platelet count measured by Sysmex XT-2000iV in dogs, cats, and horses. Vet Clin Pathol 2016;45:444–9.

17. Barton MH, Morris DD, Crowe N, et al. Hemostatic indices in healthy foals from birth to one month of age. J Vet Diagn Invest 1995;7:380–5.

18. Darien BJ, Carleton C, Kurdowska A, et al. Haemostasis and antithrombin III in the full-term newborn foal. Comp Haematol Internat 1991;1:161–5.

19. Piccione G, Arfuso F, Quartuccio M, et al. Age-related developmental clotting profile and platelet aggregation in foals over the first month of life. J Equine Vet Sci 2015;35:89–94.

20. Armengou L, Monreal L, Tarancon I, et al. Plasma D-dimer concentration in sick newborn foals. J Vet Intern Med 2008;22:411–7.

21. Watts AE, Fubini SL, Todhunter RJ, et al. Comparison of plasma and peritoneal indices of fibrinolysis between foals and adult horses with and without colic. Am J Vet Res 2011;72:1535–40.

22. Bauer JE. Normal blood chemistry. In: Koterba A, Drummond W, Kosch P, editors. Equine clinical neonatology. Philadelphia: Lea and Febiger; 1990. p. 602–14.

23. Stoneham SJ, Palmer L, Cash R, et al. Measurement of serum amyloid A in the neonatal foal using a latex agglutination immunoturbidimetric assay: determination of the normal range, variation with age and response to disease. Equine Vet J 2001;33:599–603.

24. Bauer JE, Harvey JW, Asquith RL, et al. Clinical chemistry reference values of foals during the first year of life. Equine Vet J 1984;16:361–3.

25. Dunkel B, Palmer JE, Olson KN, et al. Uroperitoneum in 32 foals: influence of intravenous fluid therapy, infection, and sepsis. J Vet Intern Med 2005;19:889–93.

26. Kablack KA, Embertson RM, Bernard WV, et al. Uroperitoneum in the hospitalised equine neonate: retrospective study of 31 cases, 1988-1997. Equine Vet J 2000; 32:505–8.

27. Axon JE, Palmer JE. Clinical pathology of the foal. Vet Clin North Am Equine Pract 2008;24:357–85.

28. Tennent-Brown B. Blood lactate measurement and interpretation in critically ill equine adults and neonates. Vet Clin North Am Equine Pract 2014;30:399–413, viii.

29. Sheahan BJ, Wilkins PA, Lascola KM, et al. The area under the curve of L-lactate in neonatal foals from birth to 14 days of age. J Vet Emerg Crit Care (San Antonio) 2016;26:305–9.

30. Chaney KP, Holcombe SJ, Schott IIHC, et al. Spurious hypercreatinemia: 28 neonatal foals (2000–2008). J Vet Emerg Crit Care (San Antonio) 2010;20:244–9.

31. Bernard WV, Hewlett L, Cudd T, et al. Historical factors, clinicopathologic findings, clinical features, and outcome of equine neonates presenting with or developing signs of central nervous system disease. Amer Assoc Equine Pract Proc of the Annual Convention 1995;41:222–4.

32. Feijó LS, Curcio BR, Pazinato FM, et al. Hematological and biochemical indicators of maturity in foals and their relation to the placental features. Pesqui Vet Bras 2018;38:1232–8.

33. Barton MH, LeRoy BE. Serum bile acids concentrations in healthy and clinically Ill neonatal foals. J Vet Intern Med 2007;21:508–13.

34. Bauer JE, Asquith RL, Kivipelto J. Serum biochemical indicators of liver function in neonatal foals. Am J Vet Res 1989;50:2037–41.

35. Wong RJ, Bhutani VK. Pathogenesis and etiology of unconjugated hyperbilirubine-mia in the newborn. In: Abrams SA, Rand EB, editors. UpToDate; 2015. Accessed June 14, 2019.

36. D'Alessandro AG, Casamassima D, Palazzo M, et al. Values of energetic, proteic and hepatic serum profiles in neonatal foals of the Martina Franca donkey breed. Macedonian J Anim Sci 2012;2:213–7.

37. Gossett KA, French DD. Effect of age on liver enzyme activities in serum of healthy quarter horses. Am J Vet Res 1984;45:354–6.

38. Haggett EF, Magdesian KG, Kass PH. Clinical implications of high liver enzyme activities in hospitalized neonatal foals. J Am Vet Med Assoc 2011;239:661–7.

39. Hank AM, Hoffmann WE, Sanecki RK, et al. Quantitative determination of equine alkaline phosphatase isoenzymes in foal and adult serum. J Vet Intern Med 1993; 7:20–4.

40. Breuhaus BA. Thyroid function and dysfunction in term and premature equine ne-onates. J Vet Intern Med 2014;28:1301–9.

41. Irvine CHG, Evans MJ. Postnatal changes in total and free thyroxine and triiodo-thyronine in foal serum. J Reprod Fertil Suppl 1975;(23):709–15.

42. Murray MJ, Luba NK. Plasma gastrin and somatostatin, and serum thyroxine (T4), triiodothyronine (T3), reverse triiodothyronine (rT3) and cortisol concentrations in foals from birth to 28 days of age. Equine Vet J 1993;25:237–9.

43. Chen CL, Riley AM. Serum thyroxine and triiodothyronine concentrations in neonatal foals and mature horses. Am J Vet Res 1981;42:1415–7.

44. Himler M, Hurcombe SD, Griffin A, et al. Presumptive nonthyroidal illness syn-drome in critically ill foals. Equine Vet J Suppl 2012;(41):43–7.

45. Pirrone A, Panzani S, Govoni N, et al. Thyroid hormone concentrations in foals affected by perinatal asphyxia syndrome. Theriogenology 2013;80:624–9.

46. Hart KA, Barton MH, Norton NA, et al. Hypothalamic-pituitary-adrenal axis assessment in healthy term neonatal foals utilizing a paired low dose/high dose ACTH stimulation test. J Vet Intern Med 2009;23:344–51.

47. Ousey JC, Turnbull C, Allen WR, et al. Effects of manipulating intrauterine growth on post natal adrenocortical development and other parameters of maturity in neonatal foals. Equine Vet J 2004;36:616–21.

48. Silver M, Fowden AL, Knox J, et al. Sympathoadrenal and other responses to hy-poglycaemia in the young foal. J Reprod Fertil Suppl 1987;35:607–14.

49. Bousquet-Melou A, Formentini E, Picard-Hagen N, et al. The adrenocorticotropin stimulation test: contribution of a physiologically based model developed in horse for its interpretation in different pathophysiological situations encountered in man. Endocrinology 2006;147:4281–91.

50. Wong DM, Vo DT, Alcott CJ, et al. Adrenocorticotropic hormone stimulation tests in healthy foals from birth to 12 weeks of age. Can J Vet Res 2009;73:65–72.

51. Hart KA, Barton MH, Ferguson DC, et al. Serum free cortisol fraction in healthy and septic neonatal foals. J Vet Intern Med 2011;25:345–55.

52. Hart KA, Dirikolu L, Ferguson DC, et al. Daily endogenous cortisol production and hydrocortisone pharmacokinetics in adult horses and neonatal foals. Am J Vet Res 2012;73:68–75.

53. Madigan JE, Haggettt EF, Pickles KJ, et al. Allopregnanolone infusion induced neurobehavioural alterations in a neonatal foal: is this a clue to the pathogenesis of neonatal maladjustment syndrome? Equine Vet J Suppl 2012;(41):109–12.

54. Dembek KA, Timko KJ, Johnson LM, et al. Steroids, steroid precursors, and neuroactive steroids in critically ill equine neonates. Vet J 2017;225:42–9.
55. Magdesian KG. Monitoring the critically ill equine patient. Vet Clin North Am Equine Pract 2004;20:11–39.
56. Madigan JE, Thomas WP, Backus KQ, et al. Mixed venous blood gases in recumbent and upright positions in foals from birth to 14 days of age. Equine Vet J 1992;24:399–401.
57. Green LG, Mayhew IG. Neurologic disorders. In: Koterba A, Drummond W, Kosch P, editors. Equine clinical neonatology. Philadelphia: Lea and Febiger; 1990. p. 496–530.
58. Furr MO, Bender H. Cerebrospinal fluid variables in clinically normal foals from birth to 42 days of age. Am J Vet Res 1994;55:781–4.
59. Behrens E, Parraga ME, Nassiff A, et al. Reference values of peritoneal fluid from healthy foals. J Equine Vet Sci 1990;10:348–52.
60. Brewer BD, Clement SF, Lotz WS, et al. Renal clearance, urinary excretion of endogenous substances, and urinary diagnostic indices in healthy neonatal foals. J Vet Intern Med 1991;5:28–33.
61. Hostetter SJ, Clark SK, Gilbertie JM, et al. Age-related variation in the cellular composition of equine bronchoalveolar lavage fluid. Vet Clin Pathol 2017;46: 344–53.

Airway Diagnostics
Bronchoalveolar Lavage, Tracheal Wash, and Pleural Fluid

Laurent L. Couetil, DVM, PhD[a],*, Craig A. Thompson, DVM[b]

KEYWORDS

- Bronchoalveolar lavage • Tracheal wash • Equine asthma • Pulmonary
- Respiratory • Cytology

KEY POINTS

- Tracheal wash is preferred for the diagnosis of infectious pulmonary diseases.
- Bronchoalveolar lavage is preferred for the diagnosis of equine asthma (ie, inflammatory airway disease and recurrent airway obstruction).
- Fluid samples should be processed as soon as possible. If a short delay (<8 hours) is anticipated, the sample should be refrigerated or placed on ice. A delay of up to 48 hours may be acceptable if the sample is refrigerated.
- Diff-Quik does not stain mast cell granules reliably. Leishman, Wright-Giemsa, and May-Grünwald Giemsa are more appropriate stains.
- Cut-off values for BAL differential cell counts in healthy adult are: neutrophils 5% or less, eosinophils 1% or less, and mast cells 2% or less.

INTRODUCTION

Cytologic analysis and microbial culture of airway secretions and pleural fluid are invaluable for proper diagnosis and to help guide therapy of horses with respiratory disease. The most common techniques used to obtain respiratory secretions are tracheal wash (TW) and bronchoalveolar lavage (BAL). In cases of pleural effusion, collection of pleural fluid by thoracocentesis may yield a diagnosis and be part of treatment (pleural drainage).

Clinical research over the last decade has greatly enhanced our understanding of airway cytologic and microbiologic findings, in particular regarding the diagnosis of equine asthma that encompasses inflammatory airway disease (mild to moderate

[a] Department of Veterinary Clinical Sciences, Purdue University College of Veterinary Medicine, 625 Harrison Street, West Lafayette, IN 47907-2026, USA; [b] Department of Comparative Pathobiology, Purdue University College of Veterinary Medicine, 725 Harrison Street, West Lafayette, IN 47907-2027, USA
* Corresponding author.
E-mail address: couetill@purdue.edu

Vet Clin Equine 36 (2020) 87–103
https://doi.org/10.1016/j.cveq.2019.12.006
0749-0739/20/© 2019 Elsevier Inc. All rights reserved.

vetequine.theclinics.com

asthma) and recurrent airway obstruction (severe asthma). This is in part due to the availability of instrumentation allowing TW and BAL to be easily and safely performed in the field. As with any diagnostic test, it is important to understand the indications for each test and factors that may affect results, such as contamination or artifacts of collection, sample processing mistakes, and how these factors may affect interpretation. Proper technical skills and knowledge of potential sources of errors will greatly decrease the risk of making incorrect conclusions. Importantly, we need to acknowledge that proper test interpretation has to be made in light of detailed historical information and clinical examination of the patient.

INDICATIONS

The main indication for a TW is diagnosis of localized infectious diseases (bacterial, fungal, or viral) of the lower respiratory tract, such as bronchopneumonia, pleuropneumonia, or lung abscess. Collection of BAL fluid is most useful to diffuse lung disease, such as equine asthma (inflammatory airway disease or recurrent airway obstruction), exercise-induced pulmonary hemorrhage, and certain infectious diseases (eg, equine herpesvirus-5). Thoracocentesis is performed for diagnostic and therapeutic purposes in cases of pleural effusion or pneumothorax. It should be noted that in cases of pleuropneumonia, it is recommended to collect both TW and pleural fluid for bacterial culture to improve odds of isolating etiologic agents.[1]

When to Choose Tracheal Wash or Bronchoalveolar Lavage for the Diagnosis of Respiratory Disease

Cases of infectious lung disease, such as bacterial pneumonia, often lead to focal (eg, cranioventral lung with pneumonia) or multifocal disease and affected areas are often adjacent to unaffected areas. Secretions originating from affected lung segments eventually collect in the trachea. In these cases, cytologic analysis and microbiological culture of TW fluid is likely to yield an etiologic diagnosis. In contrast, fluid collected by BAL is only representative of the lung region distal to the bronchus where the tube or endoscope was wedged (usually the right caudal lung lobe with blind placement). Even with endoscopic guidance, it is difficult to follow airways down to an affected lung segment. As a result, it is common to obtain BAL samples with normal cytologic findings from horses with pulmonary infection.[2] In cases of diffuse lung disease, such as equine asthma, BAL fluid cytologic results correlate well with lung inflammation histologically, with the exception of some severe cases that may show relatively few BAL neutrophils compared with the severity of lung tissue inflammation.[3] Consequently, those horses with severe equine asthma but BAL neutrophilia of less than 20% are considered to have paucigranulocytic asthma.

In cases of uncertain cause, it is best to perform both tests to maximize diagnostic yield. If both diagnostic techniques are used, TW is performed first to avoid cross-contamination.

Cut-Off Values for the Diagnosis of Equine Asthma with Bronchoalveolar Lavage and Tracheal Wash

Bronchoalveolar fluid typically consists of a mixture of pulmonary macrophages and lymphocytes. Recommended cut-offs for BAL fluid cytologic results in healthy horses include a total nucleated cell count (TNCC) of 530 cells/μL or less, neutrophils of 5% or less, eosinophils of 1% or less, and metachromatic (mast) cells of 2% or less.[4] Increased BAL neutrophil and mast cell percentages has been associated with poor performance in racehorses and evidence-based cut-off values for mild equine asthma are greater than 5% neutrophils and greater than 2% mast cells.[5] Increased BAL eosinophils have been associated with airway hyperreactivity and poor performance; however, cut-off values for a diagnosis of mild to moderate asthma based on eosinophil percentages have not been validated yet.[6] Relative cell counts do change with age with foals experiencing a decrease in the proportion of alveolar macrophages and increase in lymphocytes during the first year of life.[7]

Normal TW fluid should contain mucus, a predominance of pulmonary alveolar macrophages (40%–80%), variable numbers of epithelial cells depending on the sample collection technique (1%–50%), and lower numbers of neutrophils (<20%), lymphocytes (<10%), and eosinophils (<1%).[8–11] Mast cells are more likely to be detected in BAL than TW samples and are not usually seen in the latter.[12] Some studies suggest that TW neutrophils of greater than 20% is consistent with equine asthma.[9] However, collection of BAL is considered more appropriate, in conjunction with history and clinical signs, to help differentiate mild, moderate, and severe forms of equine asthma.[4]

The correlation between TW and BAL neutrophilia varies between studies ranging from poor ($r \leq 0.1$ or $\kappa < 0.2$; $n = 202$)[13–15] to moderate ($r = 0.67$ or $\kappa = 0.65$; $n = 154$).[9] These results mean that a different diagnosis may have been reached based on TW or BAL interpretation in at least 17% to 37% of horses. Otherwise, studies have reported weak to no correlation between the percentage of macrophages, lymphocytes, mast cells and eosinophils in TW and BAL.[9,12,14]

SAMPLE COLLECTION
Tracheal Wash

- There are 2 main techniques to collect tracheal secretions: (1) Transcutaneous catheterization in the mid-cervical region (transtracheal wash [TTW]; **Table 1**) [https://youtu.be/gWRz-ecjGUs], and (2) through the working channel of an endoscope (TW; **Table 2**) [https://youtu.be/PuhvtmXCGZ4]. The transcutaneous route is the most economical method and it allows bypassing of potential upper airway contamination of the sample. However, this method carries a risk of subcutaneous abscess formation at the puncture site because of seeding of tissue with infectious agents as the sampling catheter and needle are withdrawn. Otherwise, both the TW and TTW methods are considered similar regarding cytologic and bacteriologic findings.[8]
- Potential complications
  - TTW: Pharyngeal contamination may occur if the needle and catheter were directed upward or if the horse coughed during the procedure. Cutting off the catheter at the needle tip and loss into the airways is possible, particularly when the catheter is pulled out through the needle. Usually, the catheter is rapidly coughed out. Local cellulitis or abscess formation is particularly common with bacterial respiratory diseases. Subcutaneous emphysema at the incision site is uncommon. Tracheal trauma resulting in hemorrhage or a damaged tracheal ring with subsequent chondroma formation are rare complications.
  - TW via endoscope: Pharyngeal contamination commonly occurs if the horse coughs during the procedure. It may be difficult to aspirate fluid owing to thick secretions. Choosing a catheter with a larger lumen helps, as does infusing additional sterile solution to unplug the catheter followed by gentle aspiration. Direct aspiration of tracheal secretions via the instrument channel of the endoscope will result in contamination from proximal airways and will be inappropriate for microbiologic culture. If TW is performed to investigate nonseptic respiratory disease then, infusion and aspiration of sterile fluid using a sterile single-lumen catheter via the working channel of the endoscope is acceptable.

Table 1	
TTW procedure	
Instrumentation and supplies	1. Sterile 10-gauge needle and sterile No. 7F (2.3-mm OD) polyethylene catheter (>50 cm long) or 12-gauge needle with 5F (1.67-mm OD) PE catheter. 2. Alternatively, several commercial TTW kits are available.[a] 3. Clippers. 4. Sedation if deemed necessary or twitch. 5. No. 15 surgical blade. 6. 35 mL sterile syringe. 7. Sterile isotonic saline solution (100 mL). 8. 10 mL of 2% lidocaine. 9. Sterile gloves. 10. Tube with EDTA (purple top) for cytology and dry, sterile tube (red top) or microbiologic transport system for culture.
Procedure	1. Proper restraint: The animal should be sedated (eg, xylazine or detomidine) or nose-twitched. Consider additional pain and cough control with butorphanol tartrate (0.01–0.02 mg/kg, IV). 2. Identification of anatomic landmarks by palpating tracheal rings over the ventral aspect of the trachea in mid to distal third of the neck. 3. Clip selected area (10 × 10 cm) and sterilely prepare it. 4. Inject lidocaine subcutaneously over the site on midline (2–3 mL) and then an additional 5–10 mL injected in the soft tissue between skin and trachea and a final scrub is performed. 5. Make a small stab incision with a No. 15 blade. 6. The trachea is stabilized with one hand and the large bore needle is inserted into the trachea between 2 tracheal rings with bevel downward. After penetrating the trachea, the needle is directed downward and held tightly against the neck. 7. The catheter is inserted through the needle into the trachea for a distance of approximately 30–40 cm to reach thoracic inlet. There should no resistance when passing the catheter and air should be easily aspirated from it without creating any vacuum. 8. A 20–30 mL bolus of sterile isotonic solution is then injected rapidly through the catheter and immediately aspirated while the catheter position is adjusted to allow fluid retrieval. The horse's head should be kept elevated to prevent movement of fluid inside the trachea between the thoracic inlet and nasopharynx, thereby, minimizing the risk of upper airway contamination during the procedure. Only 2–3 mL of fluid is needed for cytology and bacteriology. Once an adequate sample has been obtained (mucus flecks floating), the catheter is removed, then the needle. 9. The sample should be place in dry tube (red top) for aerobic/anaerobic culture of bacteria if indicated. Another aliquot should place in EDTA tube (purple top) for cytology. 10. The neck incision may be covered with topical application of antiseptic ointment over gauze and secured with an elastic adhesive bandage (no more than 24 h).

Abbreviations: IV, intravenous; OD, outer diameter.
  [a] Example of transtracheal commercial kits:
• Jorgensen Labs – Equine TW Kit: https://www.jorvet.com/product/equine-tracheal-wash-kit/
• Mila - Large Animal Trans-TW Kit/TTL: http://www.milainternational.com/index.php/products/trans-tracheal-wash-kit/large-animal-trans-tracheal-wash-kit-ttl.html
• Patterson - TW Kit with Stiff Catheter: https://www.pattersonvet.com/Supplies/ProductFamilyDetails/PIF_34116.

Table 2 TW by endoscopy	
Instrumentation and supplies	1. Minimum length of endoscope 100 cm (optimum 120–150 cm). 2. Sterile double or triple lumen catheter. 3. 35 mL sterile syringe. 4. Sterile isotonic saline solution.
Procedure	1. The animal should be tranquilized (eg, xylazine: 0.3–0.5 mg/kg, IV) or a nose twitch applied. TW may be done without sedation as long as the horse is properly restrained by nose twitch or other method deemed appropriate. This approach is often considered in performance horses to avoid drug residues before a competition. 2. The catheter is advanced in the endoscope's instrument channel until it reaches the tip. 3. The endoscope is passed through proximal airways until the midcervical trachea. 4. The catheter is exteriorized and the sterile inner tubing(s) deployed. 5. A 20–30 mL bolus of sterile isotonic solution is then injected rapidly through the catheter and immediately aspirated while positioning catheter tip in the tracheal puddle. A minimum of 2 mL of fluid is needed for cytology and bacteriology. 6. The sample should be cultured for aerobic/anaerobic bacteria if indicated. Another aliquot should be submitted for cytology (prepare directly air-dried slides or submit sample in syringe/EDTA tube to laboratory).

- Mila - TW/aspiration catheters: http://www.milainternational.com/index.php/products/trans-tracheal-wash-kit/tracheal-wash-aspiration-catheters.html
  - Single-lumen – Single-lumen catheter with a female luer lock for medication delivery and sampling at any endoscope accessible site. To maintain sterility during placement, these sets contain a glycol plug. - Item Number - EDC190, EDC220, and EDC400–2.3 mm OD
  - Double or triple lumen – Two- and 3-lumen sampling catheters enable a sterile specimen retrieval via an endoscope. To maintain sterility during placement, these sets contain a glycol plug in the outer catheter. Once placed, the inner catheter is advanced for retrieval of the sterile specimen.
    - Two-stage/double-lumen item numbers - EMAC700, EMAC700 L (1.8 mm OD)
    - Triple-stage/triple-lumen item number - EMAC800 (2.3 mm OD)

Abbreviation: IV, intravenously.

Bronchoalveolar Lavage

- There are 2 main techniques to perform a BAL: Using an endoscope (**Table 3**) or performing it blindly using a BAL catheter (**Table 4**) [https://youtu.be/qwZOAZ5-xFM].
- Procedure
  - Pretreatment of horses with severe equine asthma (recurrent airway obstruction or heaves) with a bronchodilator (eg, inhaled albuterol 1 μg/kg) may help to increase BAL fluid volume yield during the procedure.[16]
  - A volume of 250 mL of warm sterile saline solution is infused (1 bolus for 250 mL pressurized fluid bag or 5 × 50 mL syringes). BAL fluid yield may be higher when using gentle suction with 60-mL syringes as compared with suction.[17] Greater infusion volume may also be used (eg, 500 mL); however, the extra dilution needs to be taken in consideration when interpreting cell counts; therefore, it is important to always use the same infusion volume.[18]
  - Average BAL fluid return is 40% to 70% of the infused volume. A lower return may be anticipated in horses with severe airway inflammation.

Table 3 BAL procedure via endoscopy	
Instrumentation and supplies	1. A 180–200 cm long minimum, 8–10 mm diameter endoscope. 2. Use 250 mL of warm sterile isotonic saline solution, pressurized infusion set, and suction pump. Alternatively, use 60-mL sterile syringes to administer and retrieve fluid. 3. Use 60 mL of warm lidocaine solution (10 mL of 2% lidocaine in 50 mL of sterile solution). 4. Bucket of ice.
Technique	1. The animal should be tranquilized (eg, xylazine: 0.4–0.8 mg/kg, IV) and a nose twitch applied. Butorphanol administration (0.01–0.02 mg/kg IV) helps to decrease coughing. 2. Pass the endoscope through the nose and instill diluted lidocaine solution onto the larynx (5–10 mL) via the working channel. Advance the endoscope into the trachea and instill lidocaine solution as needed if the horse is coughing excessively. This technique is especially needed when at the level of the carina (10–20 mL) and then, during advancement of the endoscope inside bronchi (4–5 mL at each step) until it becomes wedged in a distal airway. 3. Infuse sterile solution rapidly (eg, using pressurized bag or preloaded 60-mL syringes) while maintaining the endoscope wedged. 4. Suction BAL fluid immediately by hand with 60 mL syringes or via a suction pump (<300 mm Hg). 5. Pool BAL fluid from all syringes in a container kept on ice until processing (within 4 h of collection).

Abbreviation: IV, intravenously.

- Potential complications
  - Poor sample return (<20 mL) or clear fluid with no foam (surfactant) suggest incorrect tube placement (eg, tube retroflexion, improper wedge, or placement in the esophagus). The tube should be removed and the procedure repeated. Low sample return with little foam is also common in horses with severe asthma. In such cases, pretreatment with bronchodilator may improve yield and instilling a second fluid bolus (250 mL) is helpful to obtain at least 40 to 50 mL of BAL fluid (tube dead space of approximately 20 mL).
  - Excessive coughing: Coughing is expected as the tube is advanced into the airways and wedged. However, it usually stops promptly as saline is infused. Therefore, lavage fluid should be administered as soon as possible after wedging and cuff inflation. Rarely, a horse may cough continuously during the procedure and, in such cases, the procedure should be aborted.
  - Local, mild neutrophilic inflammation develops but spontaneously resolves within 48 hours. Normal training in performance horses may resume the next day. Transient pyrexia is very rare and usually resolves within 24 hours without treatment.

Thoracocentesis

- The procedure is easily done on standing horses restrained in stocks and with sedation if appropriate (**Table 5**). Thoracic ultrasound examination is invaluable to identify the extent of pleural effusion and important landmarks, such as the heart and lung, to optimize positioning of the thoracocentesis needle. Alternatively, the extent of the fluid line may be determined by thoracic auscultation and percussion. The equine mediastinum is fenestrated cranioventrally, allowing fluid to migrate from one side to another. However, communication between both

Table 4 BAL procedure with a catheter	
Instrumentation and supplies	1. A 240–300 cm long, 10 mm diameter bronchoalveolar catheter with cuff.[a] 2. 5 × 60-mL sterile syringes. 3. 250 mL of warm sterile isotonic saline solution. 4. 60 ml of warm lidocaine solution (10 mL of 2% lidocaine in 50 mL sterile solution). 5. 3-way stopcock valve. 6. Lidocaine viscous solution (2%)[b] is optional. 7. Bucket of ice.
Technique	1. The animal should be tranquilized (eg, xylazine: 0.4–0.8 mg/kg, IV) and a nose twitch applied. Butorphanol administration (0.01–0.02 mg/kg IV) helps decrease coughing. 2. Fill BAL catheter dead space with diluted lidocaine solution and close off stopcock valve. 3. Premeasure and mark the catheter to indicate approximate distance between nares and larynx (lateral canthus) and carina (point of the shoulder). 4. Apply lidocaine viscous solution (2%) on the tip of the BAL catheter. 5. Pass the BAL tube through the nose until in front of the larynx. Instill diluted lidocaine solution onto the larynx (5–10 mL) to decrease coughing. 6. Advance the BAL catheter into the trachea. Extending the head and neck facilitates passage. Shaking the trachea and feeling the tube bumping against the wall confirms proper placement. Instill 10–20 mL lidocaine solution onto the carina. 7. Continue to advance the catheter until it becomes wedged in a distal airway. Proper wedging is indicated by a slight increase in resistance as the instrument is advanced. Inflate the tube cuff with air. 8. Infuse sterile solution rapidly using preloaded 60-mL syringes (or pressurized 250 mL fluid bag) while maintaining the catheter wedged. 9. Suction BAL fluid immediately but gently by hand with 60-mL syringes. 10. Pool the BAL fluid from all syringes in a container kept on ice until processing (within 4 h of collection).

Abbreviation: IV, intravenously.
[a] Example of commercially available BAL catheters:
• Mila – Large Animal BAL catheter: http://www.milainternational.com/index.php/large-animal-broncho-alveolar-lavage-catheter-bal.html
  ○ 10 mm OD, 2.5 mm ID, 240 or 300 cm long, 50 mL distal balloon
• Jorgensen Labs – Broncho-alveolar Lavage catheter: https://www.jorvet.com/product/broncho-alveolar-lavage-catheter/
  ○ 10 mm OD (30 Fr), 240 cm long, 10 mL cuff.
[b] Lidocaine HCl viscous solution 2%, 100 ml bottle.

hemithoraces is often sealed in inflammatory and infectious processes and collection of pleural fluid from both sides is recommended to maximize diagnostic utility.
• Potential complications
  ○ Pneumothorax or hemothorax
  ○ Local cellulitis or abscess at the insertion site

HANDLING AND PREPARATION OF BRONCHOALVEOLAR LAVAGE FLUID

The interpretation of BAL cytology requires expertise and experience; therefore, it is not recommended that practitioners attempt to read their own slides. However, it is

Table 5 Thoracocentesis procedure	
Instrumentation and supplies	1. Sterile 3³/₄ in (9-cm long) stainless steel teat cannula or sterile 14 gauge– 5¹/₄ in (13 cm long) Teflon catheter. Teat cannula is preferred because the blunt tip will minimize damage to blood vessels and avoid lung laceration. 2. IV extension set (30 in [75 cm]) and a 3-way stopcock valve. 3. Clippers. 4. Sedation if deemed necessary or twitch. 5. No. 15 surgical blade. 6. 20 mL sterile syringe. 7. 10–20 mL of 2% lidocaine with 1½ in (20 gauge) needle. 8. Sterile gloves. 9. Tube with EDTA (purple top) for cytology and dry, sterile tube (red top) or microbiologic transport system for culture.
Procedure	1. Proper restraint: The animal should be sedated (eg, xylazine or detomidine). 2. Identification of anatomic landmarks by ultrasound imaging (preferable) or if conducting the procedure blindly: (a) right side in the 6th–7th intercostal spaces and approximately one hand width (10 cm) above the olecranon; b) left side, in the 6th–9th intercostal spaces and 5 cm above the olecranon. 3. Clip selected area (10 × 10 cm) and sterilely prepare it. 4. Inject lidocaine subcutaneously (4–5 mL) starting 2–3 cm caudal to the insertion site and then progressing cranially over intercostal space. Redirect syringe and needle perpendicularly to body wall on the cranial edge of the rib and inject an additional 5–10 mL in the intercostal muscle and parietal pleura. The latter is particular sensitive. Care should be taken to avoid damaging blood vessels and nerves running immediately caudal to each rib. 5. Make a small stab incision with a No. 15 blade 2–3 cm caudal to intercostal space. 6. The cannula is first connected to extension tubing and a 3-way stop cock in the closed position. The cannula is carefully inserted through the stab incision at a shallow angle while pointing the tip cranially and tunneling under the skin until it reaches the cranial aspect of the rib. 7. The cannula is then rotated perpendicularly to the chest wall and pushed through the chest wall. Passage into the pleural space will be felt as a sudden loss of resistance to advancement of the cannula. At this point, the 3-way stop cock is opened to allow drainage of pleural fluid. If fluid does not drain spontaneously, redirect the cannula or apply gentle suction with a syringe. 8. The sample should be place in dry tube (red top) for aerobic/anaerobic culture of bacteria if indicated. Another aliquot should place in EDTA tube (purple top) for cytology. 9. Both sides of the thorax should be tapped if a bilateral condition exists. 10. The thoracic incision may be covered with topical application of antiseptic ointment over gauze and secured with an elastic adhesive bandage (no more than 24 h).
Complications	1. Pneumothorax or hemothorax. 2. Local cellulitis or abscess at the insertion site.

Abbreviation: IV, intravenously.

important to process and submit BAL appropriately to optimize cell preservation and interpretation by the laboratory. Ideally, the sample should be processed immediately; however, logistically, this is often not feasible. Storage time should be minimized for best cell preservation and restricting bacterial growth. If a short delay (<8 hours) is anticipated, refrigeration or placing the sample on ice is ideal. A delay of up to 48 hours is acceptable if the sample is refrigerated.

If large particles or chunks are seen on gross examination of the BAL, these can be removed by passing the fluid through gauze, although this is usually done in the laboratory. An aliquot of well-mixed BAL should be submitted to the laboratory in EDTA (5–10 mL) to prevent cell clumping or the entire sample can be submitted in a sealed container kept cool if processing in-house. Do not add formalin or alcohol because they change the cell morphologic features dramatically. If submitting the sample to a referral laboratory, it should shipped overnight on an icepack in an insulated container, ideally with a smear prepared from the fresh fluid. To make a smear from the cell pellet, an aliquot of BAL (eg, 20 mL) can be processed using a table-top centrifuge (eg, around $328 \times g$ for 6 minutes). The supernatant is decanted with subsequent resuspension of the pellet with remaining fluid (<0.5 mL). Ten microliters (or a small drop) of equine serum can be added to the resuspended pellet to help preserve cells.[19] The pellet is then smeared onto a slide using the traditional technique for making a blood smear and air dried quickly (eg, fan or hair dryer). This technique produces smears that are adequately diagnostic for neutrophilic pulmonary disease; however, the cells do not spread as well as smears made with a cytocentrifuge in referral clinical pathology laboratories and it is difficult to differentiate macrophages and lymphocytes.[19] Most laboratories will make their own smears, but submitting smears of fresh BAL helps with interpretation owing to storage-associated changes in cells. In this case, it is recommended to let the laboratory know how the smear was made. Cytocentrifugation is ideal for BAL cytologic analysis, but the equipment is expensive and typically only available in laboratories.

Most clinical pathologic laboratories prefer to use their own equipment to stain slides, so submission of unstained smears is preferable. If in-house staining is desired, rapid Romanowsky stains such as Diff-Quik are widely available and convenient. A drawback to these stains is the lack of, or poor, staining of mast cell granules, leading to gross underestimation of the mast cell percentage.[20] To avoid this problem, it is recommended that other stains, such as Leishman's, Wright-Giemsa, May-Grünwald, or Giemsa, be used.[20]

The TNCC and red blood cell (RBC) count in BAL can be determined with a hemocytometer (some laboratories will first filter the BAL before doing counts and smears). Directions are available from the manufacturer and involve mixing the fluid with a diluent (can lyse erythrocytes), loading the hemocytometer, counting nucleated cells within a prescribed area, then applying a mathematical formula to account for the dilution and volume analyzed. If a sample is free from mucus strands and grossly visible particles, it can be evaluated with an automated hematology analyzer to produce a TNCC and RBC count; however, no studies have been performed to evaluate this practice and it may be analyzer dependent. For example, manual and automated nucleated cell counts correlate poorly in pleural and peritoneal fluid samples with a TNCC of less than 1000/μL[21] and in most BAL samples, the TNCC is less than 500/μL. The TNCC and proportion of cell types can be influenced by the volume of wash fluid needed to obtain the sample. One study showed a lower percentage of neutrophils when 500 mL versus 250 mL of saline was used for collection, which could affect interpretation.[18] Therefore, it is important to always use the same volume of fluid to perform a BAL (between 250 and 500 mL).[4]

HANDLING AND PREPARATION OF TRACHEAL WASH FLUID

Laboratories may prepare TW fluid differently for cytologic analysis. In some laboratories, large particles or chunks that are seen on gross examination of the fluid may be removed by passing the fluid through gauze, followed by preparation of cytocentrifuged smears. In other laboratories, direct or centrifuged smears (using a regular table top centrifuge) are prepared from the fluid, depending on gross turbidity, using the squash technique between 2 slides. Slides are then air dried quickly, because TW fluid contain mucus and dry slowly. Once smears have been prepared, they are stained for microscopic examination as described elsewhere in this article. Alternatively, TW fluid may be shipped to a clinical pathology laboratory in an EDTA tube accompanied with unstained smears of fresh samples as indicated elsewhere in this article.

EVALUATION OF AIRWAY SAMPLES

Evaluation of BAL fluid smears involves performing a nucleated differential cell count, morphologic evaluation of cells and an assessment of background components. Pooling samples from each side or from different aliquots does not affect diagnosis of equine asthma.[22] If smears are made from the pellet of a centrifuged BAL sample, as indicated, and cellularity allows, a traditional 400- or 500-cell differential can be performed in areas where morphologic features can be adequately evaluated. Using cytocentrifuge preparations allows the use of a 5-field method, which involves performing a nucleated differential cell count on 5 fields on a cytocentrifuge smear, provided the cells are well-preserved and readily identified (not often the case in stored samples) and if there are more than 100 cells present on a field viewed through the 50× objective (500×). With this degree of cellularity, the 5-field method is acceptable for all cells, including mast cells.[23] Cytologic assessment of TW samples does not usually include TNCC, RBC counts, or nucleated differential cell counts, but this may vary between laboratories. Rather, a subjective assessment of proportion of inflammatory cells (macrophages, which normally dominate in TW fluids, with <20% neutrophils and low numbers of lymphocytes), along with their morphologic features, and other cell types (described elsewhere in this article) is provided.

Neutrophils are not normally airway resident cells and their morphologic features can be helpful. Nondegenerate and degenerate neutrophils (**Figs. 1** and **2**) are more likely associated with sterile processes or bacterial infection, respectively.[24] Nondegenerate neutrophils look essentially the same as they do in the circulation (see **Fig. 1**). They generally have up to 5 nuclear lobes and display a condensed chromatin pattern. Aged neutrophils look similar, but can be hypersegmented (ie, >5 nuclear lobes). Often in the case of aged neutrophils, the lobes are separated by thinner than normal internuclear bridges. Seeing exclusively nondegenerate and aged neutrophils may support a nonseptic environment. Degenerate changes involve the nucleus and are visualized as karyolysis, which is an indicator of oncotic cell death. Karyolysis must be determined within an intact cell, because similar changes can be observed in nuclei that have been stripped of cytoplasm or in samples that have been stored (see **Figs. 1** and **2**). Karyorrhexis and pyknosis may represent oncosis or apoptosis and thus cannot be relied on to detect changes to the in situ environment. Macrophages are highly variable in appearance, ranging from quiescent, minimally vacuolated mononuclear cells to activated mononuclear (see **Fig. 1**) or multinucleated giant cells that are vacuolated and may contain phagocytic debris. In a fresh sample, macrophages that have phagocytized erythrocytes signal in vivo hemorrhage has occurred. With in vivo hemorrhage, the iron from the phagocytized erythrocytes will be

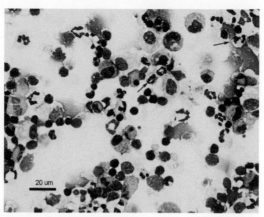

Fig. 1. Marked, mixed inflammation consisting of nondegenerate neutrophils (*arrows*), slightly activated macrophages, eosinophils (*asterisks*), and small lymphocytes in a background of lysed cells/nuclear debris and a few erythrocytes. Cytospin preparation of BAL fluid from an asthmatic horse (ie, inflammatory airway disease). Stain: Modified Wright's; original magnification, ×60 objective.

converted to hemosiderin over the course of 24 to 72 hours, yielding hemosiderophages (**Fig. 3**). Both erythrophages and hemosiderophages are key diagnostic finding in exercise-induced pulmonary hemorrhage, but are not specific for this condition (eg, can be seen with pneumonia).[25] In vitro erythrophagia may occur if there is a delay between sample acquisition and processing. Eosinophils are readily identified (see **Fig. 1**) in most airway fluids, but may hypolobulate and/or their granules stain abnormally. Lymphocytes are mostly small mature cells (see **Fig. 1**) and mast cells are normally found in BAL, but are rare in TW fluids (**Fig. 4**).

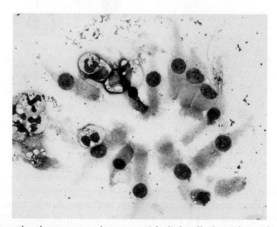

Fig. 2. Several normal columnar respiratory epithelial cells (mostly with cilia) with several mildly to moderately degenerate neutrophils, as seen by karyolysis, that is, a swollen nucleus, with chromatin that is, less condensed and may look glassy or hyalinized. A mixed population of bacteria is seen within the neutrophils. Respiratory epithelial cells may appear with and without cilia. TW from a horse with septic pneumonia. Stain: Modified Wright's; original magnification, ×100 objective.

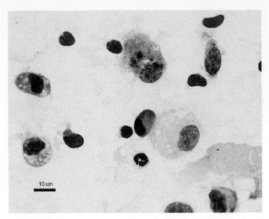

Fig. 3. Several minimally to lightly vacuolated macrophages with a single hemosiderophage containing several variably sized clumps of golden to yellow–brown aggregates of hemosiderin. Cytospin preparation of BAL fluid from a horse with exercise-induced pulmonary hemorrhage. Stain: Modified Wright's; original magnification, ×100 objective.

In addition to the inflammatory cells described, other cells can be seen within airway wash samples, including columnar (see **Figs. 2** and **4**) and goblet epithelial cells from the tracheal mucosa, squamous epithelial cells from the oropharynx (**Fig. 5**), and environmental elements (**Fig. 6**). Unremarkable respiratory epithelial cells are seen as singlets as well as in small clusters (see **Fig. 2**). Not uncommonly as a result of chronic irritation, these cells become hyperplastic (see **Fig. 4**). Squamous epithelial cells are

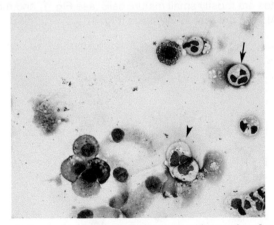

Fig. 4. Nondegenerate (*arrow*) to moderately degenerate (*arrow head*) neutrophils, a small cluster of hyperplastic (reactive) epithelial cells and a single moderately granulated mast cell (*asterisk*). A small, mixed population of bacteria are seen within neutrophils, with low numbers in the background. Mast cells are round cells that range in size from 15 to 25 μm in diameter. They have a round nucleus that typically fills half to three-quarters of the cytoplasm, which contains variable numbers of small, light to dark purple granules. Hyperplastic epithelial cells have a higher nuclear to cytoplasmic ratio than normal, darker blue cytoplasm and are more rounded to cuboidal, rather than the normal columnar shape. TW from a horse with septic pneumonia. Stain: Modified Wright's; original magnification, ×100 objective.

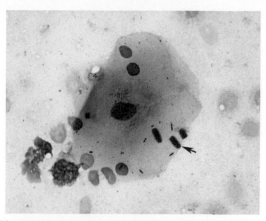

Fig. 5. A nucleated keratinized squamous epithelial cell with melanin granules and a few adherent bacteria, including *Simonsiella* sp. (*arrow*). Squamous epithelial cells are large angular cells that have blue keratinized cytoplasm with sharp, angular margins. *Simonsiella* bacteria look like a caterpillar, with the shape being derived from side-to-side, rather than end-to-end, division. TW. Stain: Modified Wright's; original magnification, ×100 objective.

occasionally seen and represent an upper airway or skin (with TTW) contaminant obtained during sample acquisition. These cells may have adherent bacteria and, in the case of oropharyngeal contamination, *Simonsiella* sp. can be seen (see **Fig. 5**). In the background as well as within or attached to macrophages, environmental contaminants that have been inhaled may be identified, such as pollen, fungal spores, and fungal elements (see **Fig. 6**). Mineralized material may reflect another inhaled environmental contaminant or an artifact of collection (precipitation of salt crystals). Finally, mucus is a common finding in TW samples (that have not been filtered) and appears as thin to moderately thick strands of dark purple material. Mucus can be seen as tortuous, corkscrew shapes known as Curschmann's spirals, particularly in cases of

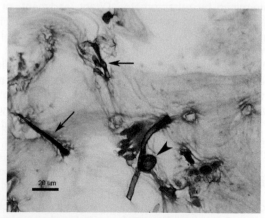

Fig. 6. A moderate amount of thick mucus strands with a variety of fungal elements (arrows), pollen (arrowhead), and debris inhaled from the environment. TW. Stain: Modified Wright's; original magnification, x100 objective.

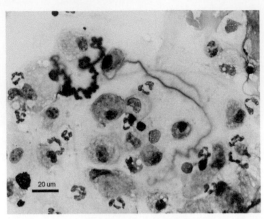

Fig. 7. Mild to moderate mixed inflammation with a large, dark, twisted Curchmann's spiral and a small amount of mucus and debris in the background. Cytospin preparation of BAL fluid from a horse with severe asthma. Stain: Modified Wright's; original magnification, ×60 objective.

chronic airway disease (**Fig. 7**). Mucus may be seen in BAL fluids when the fluid is not filtered before smears are made.

PLEURAL FLUID SAMPLE HANDLING AND PREPARATION

Pleural fluid is handled and processed similarly to airway fluids, in that both the fluid and smears made from freshly collected fluid should be submitted for cytologic evaluation. During sample acquisition, the color of the sample is noted (ie, a bloody sample throughout acquisition suggests a hemorrhagic fluid in situ). The fluid should be placed into an EDTA tube and a nonanticoagulant or red top tube, for cytologic and biochemical testing, respectively. The sample from the nonanticoagulant tube can be used for aerobic microbiologic studies; however, if available, a culturette should be used. Special transport media should be used for anaerobic microbiologic studies. In the laboratory, the color and clarity of the sample is assessed and recorded and the total protein is determined by refractometry. Direct, sediment, or cytocentrifuged smears are prepared as described elsewhere in this article for airway fluids, depending on the cellularity of the sample (ie, cytocentrifugation is preferred for low cellularity fluids). However, in a practice setting where a cytocentrifuge is not readily available, a smear of the pellet from a standard centrifuged sample will suffice. A TNCC and RBC count are usually provided and can be performed in house with a hemocytometer (if available), but most laboratories use particle counters or hematology analyzers. A study evaluating automated hematology analyzers for performing cell counts in body cavity fluids, including equine pleural fluid showed that an automated analyzer (ADVIA 120; Siemens, Munich, Germany) reliably determined the TNCC when the count was higher than 1000/μL.[21]

CYTOLOGIC EVALUATION OF PLEURAL FLUID

Pleural effusions from healthy horses should have less than 8000 nucleated cells and a total protein of less than 3.4 g/dL.[26] The cytologic profile of pleural fluid in health consists of a mixture of large mononuclear cells as well as small lymphocytes, with occasional neutrophils and rare eosinophils. The large mononuclear cells are mostly

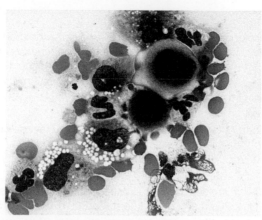

Fig. 8. Two moderately reactive mesothelial cells, with cytoplasmic blebs, and nondegenerate neutrophils and mildly reactive (vacuolated and/or phagocytic) macrophages. One of the mesothelial cells (the upper cell) is binucleated. Pleural effusion. Stain: Modified Wright's; original magnification, ×100 objective.

macrophages with a few mesothelial cells. Mesothelial cells line serosal body cavities and may appear similar to nonactivated macrophages when quiescent; however, they usually exhibit more cytoplasmic blebbing and/or a ruffled fringe around them. These cells readily become hyperplastic, often becoming darker and displaying atypia, such as binucleation and anisokaryosis, which should not be mistaken for malignancy (**Fig. 8**). Inflammatory cells within the pleural space are identical to those described in airway washings. By far, the most important is the proportion and morphologic features of neutrophils (**Fig. 9**). As indicated, degenerate neutrophils imply an underlying bacterial infection. Septic processes usually result in an increased total protein concentration, TNCC, and neutrophil percentage, and neutrophils may or may not be degenerate.

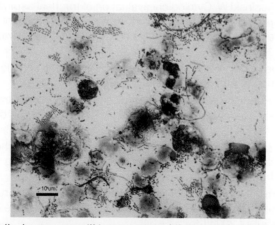

Fig. 9. Two markedly degenerate still intact neutrophils in a moderate heavy background of lysed dying cells (likely neutrophils), a few erythrocytes and large numbers of a mixed population of bacteria, consisting of cocci and variably sized rods. Pleural fluid from a horse with pleuropneumonia. Stain: Modified Wright's; original magnification ×60 objective.

REFERENCES

1. Sweeney CR, Holcombe SJ, Barningham SC, et al. Aerobic and anaerobic bacterial isolates from horses with pneumonia or pleuropneumonia and antimicrobial susceptibility patterns of the aerobes. J Am Vet Med Assoc 1991;198:839–42.
2. Rossier Y, Sweeney CR, Ziemer EL. Bronchoalveolar lavage fluid cytologic findings in horses with pneumonia or pleuropneumonia. J Am Vet Med Assoc 1991;198:1001–4.
3. Bullone M, Joubert P, Gagné A, et al. Bronchoalveolar lavage fluid neutrophilia is associated with the severity of pulmonary lesions during equine asthma exacerbations. Equine Vet J 2018;50(5):609–15. Available at: http://doi.wiley.com/10.1111/evj.12806. Accessed March 5, 2018.
4. Couëtil LI, Cardwell Jm, Gerber V, et al. Inflammatory airway disease of horses—revised consensus statement. J Vet Intern Med 2016;30:503–15.
5. Ivester KM, Couëtil LL, Moore GE. An observational study of environmental exposures, airway cytology, and performance in racing thoroughbreds. J Vet Intern Med 2018;32:1754–62.
6. Hare JE, Viel L. Pulmonary eosinophilia associated with increased airway responsiveness in young racing horses. J Vet Intern Med 1998;12:163–70.
7. Hostetter SJ, Clark SK, Gilbertie JM, et al. Age-related variation in the cellular composition of equine bronchoalveolar lavage fluid. Vet Clin Pathol 2017;46:344–53.
8. Christley RM, Hodgson DR, Rose RJ, et al. Comparison of bacteriology and cytology of tracheal fluid samples collected by percutaneous transtracheal aspiration or via an endoscope using a plugged, guarded catheter. Equine Vet J 1999;31:197–202.
9. Rossi H, Virtala A-M, Raekallio M, et al. Comparison of tracheal wash and bronchoalveolar lavage cytology in 154 horses with and without respiratory signs in a referral hospital over 2009–2015. Front Vet Sci 2018;5:61. Available at: https://www.frontiersin.org/articles/10.3389/fvets.2018.00061/full. Accessed May 1, 2019.
10. Wysocka B, Kluciński W. Cytological evaluation of tracheal aspirate and bronchoalveolar lavage fluid in comparison to endoscopic assessment of lower airways in horses with recurrent airways obstruction or inflammatory airway disease. Pol J Vet Sci 2015;18:587–97.
11. Mair TS. Value of tracheal aspirates in the diagnosis of chronic pulmonary diseases in the horse. Equine Vet J 1987;19:463–5.
12. Malikides N, Hughes KJ, Hodgson DR, et al. Comparison of tracheal aspirates and bronchoalveolar lavage in racehorses. 2. Evaluation of the diagnostic significance of neutrophil percentage. Aust Vet J 2003;81:685–7.
13. Derksen FJ, Brown CM, Sonea I, et al. Comparison of transtracheal aspirate and bronchoalveolar lavage cytology in 50 horses with chronic lung disease. Equine Vet J 1989;21:23–6.
14. Allen KJ, Tremaine WH, Franklin SH. Prevalence of inflammatory airway disease in national hunt horses referred for investigation of poor athletic performance. Equine Vet J Suppl 2006;(36):529–34.
15. Hughes K, Malikides N, Hodgson D, et al. Comparison of tracheal aspirates and bronchoalveolar lavage in racehorses 1. Evaluation of cytological stains and the percentage of mast cells and eosinophils. Aust Vet J 2003;81:681–4.

16. Varegg MS, Kløverød KM, Austnes MK, et al. The effect of single pretreatment with salbutamol on recovery of bronchoalveolar lavage fluid in horses with suspected or confirmed severe equine asthma. J Vet Intern Med 2019;33:976–80.

17. Bowser JE, Costa LRR, Rodil AU, et al. Effect of a syringe aspiration technique versus a mechanical suction technique and use of N-butylscopolammonium bromide on the quantity and quality of bronchoalveolar lavage fluid samples obtained from horses with the summer pasture endophenotype of equine asthma. Am J Vet Res 2018;79:348–55.

18. Orard M, Depecker M, Hue E, et al. Influence of bronchoalveolar lavage volume on cytological profiles and subsequent diagnosis of inflammatory airway disease in horses. Vet J 2016;207:193–5. Available at: http://www.sciencedirect.com/science/article/pii/S1090023315003974. Accessed December 1, 2015.

19. Pickles K, Pirie RS, Rhind S, et al. Cytological analysis of equine bronchoalveolar lavage fluid. Part 2: comparison of smear and cytocentrifuged preparations. Equine Vet J 2002;34:292–6.

20. Leclere M, Desnoyers M, Beauchamp G, et al. Comparison of four staining methods for detection of mast cells in equine bronchoalveolar lavage fluid. J Vet Intern Med 2006;20:377–81.

21. Gorman ME, Villarroel A, Tornquist SJ, et al. Comparison between manual and automated total nucleated cell counts using the ADVIA 120 for pleural and peritoneal fluid samples from dogs, cats, horses, and alpacas. Vet Clin Pathol 2009; 38:388–91.

22. Pickles K, Pirie RS, Rhind S, et al. Cytological analysis of equine bronchoalveolar lavage fluid. Part 1: comparison of sequential and pooled aliquots. Equine Vet J 2002;34:288–91.

23. Fernandez NJ, Hecker KG, Gilroy CV, et al. Reliability of 400-cell and 5-field leukocyte differential counts for equine bronchoalveolar lavage fluid. Vet Clin Pathol 2013;42:92–8.

24. Jocelyn NA, Wylie CE, Lean M, et al. Association of neutrophil morphology with bacterial isolates in equine tracheal wash samples. Equine Vet J 2018;50:752–8.

25. Doucet MY, Viel L. Alveolar macrophage graded hemosiderin score from bronchoalveolar lavage in horses with exercise-induced pulmonary hemorrhage and controls. J Vet Intern Med 2002;16:281–6.

26. Wagner AE, Bennett DG. Analysis of equine thoracic fluid. Vet Clin Pathol 1982; 11:13–7.

Clinical Pathology in the Adult Sick Horse

The Gastrointestinal System and Liver

SallyAnne L. DeNotta, DVM, PhD[a],*, Thomas J. Divers, DVM[b]

KEYWORDS

- Hematology • Chemistry • Enteropathy • Hepatopathy • Hyperammonemia

KEY POINTS

- Horses with acute inflammatory intestinal conditions, for example, enteritis and colitis, often present with clinical and hematologic evidence of endotoxemia, plasma volume contraction, acid-base disturbances, and electrolyte derangements.
- Horses with chronic enteropathies frequently display evidence of malabsorption and protein loss, including weight loss despite good appetite, hypoproteinemia characterized predominantly by hypoalbuminemia, and blunted glucose-absorption curves.
- Liver disease is common in horses but liver failure is uncommon.
- Liver-specific enzymes sorbitol dehydrogenase and glutamate dehydrogenase reflect hepatocellular injury, whereas γ-glutamyltransferase indicates biliary disease. Other enzymes, such as aspartate aminotransferase, lactic dehydrogenase (hepatocellular), and alkaline phosphatase (biliary), may support the diagnosis of hepatopathy, but these enzymes are not liver-specific.
- Liver function tests include conjugated and unconjugated bilirubin, ammonia, bile acids, and coagulation tests (prothrombin/partial thromboplastin times).

INTRODUCTION

The gastrointestinal tract and liver comprise key components of the equine digestive system and together have important functions in metabolism, digestion, detoxification, and synthesis. Disorders of the gastrointestinal tract and liver are common in clinical practice, whereas failure of either organ system is less common. Hematologic and biochemical analysis can be helpful for identifying organ dysfunction, narrowing down the differential diagnostic list, and, in many cases, monitoring progress and response to treatment. This article details hematologic and biochemical tests that are important

[a] Department of Large Animal Clinical Sciences, College of Veterinary Medicine, University of Florida, 2015 Southwest 16th Avenue, Gainesville, FL 32608, USA; [b] Department of Clinical Sciences, College of Veterinary Medicine, Cornell University, 144 East Avenue, Ithaca NY 14853, USA
* Corresponding author.
E-mail address: s.denotta@ufl.edu

Vet Clin Equine 36 (2020) 105–120
https://doi.org/10.1016/j.cveq.2019.11.004
0749-0739/20/© 2019 Elsevier Inc. All rights reserved.

in the evaluation of intestinal and hepatic diseases and reviews bloodwork trends frequently observed in adult horses affected by enteropathy or hepatopathy.

ACUTE GASTROINTESTINAL DISEASE

Horses with acute inflammatory intestinal conditions, for example, proximal enteritis and colitis, often present with hematologic and biochemical findings suggestive of endotoxemia (leukopenia characterized by neutropenia), plasma volume contraction (increased hematocrit, high urine-specific gravity [USG], and prerenal azotemia), and electrolyte derangements (hyponatremia, hypochloremia, and hypomagnesemia). These derangements result from intestinal inflammation and mucosal barrier disruption, leading to fluid, electrolyte, and protein loss as well as endotoxin and bacterial translocation into the blood stream. Neutropenia reflects neutrophil margination and sequestration in the intestinal tract, with left shift and toxic changes commonly observed. Strong ion acidosis characterized by hyponatremia and hyperlactatemia also is common, although a hypoproteinemic alkalosis occasionally may occur.[1] Hemoconcentration and plasma volume contraction occurs secondarily to fluid sequestration and loss via the intestines. Lower than expected total protein (especially albumin) concentration, considering the relative erythrocytosis and estimated degree of dehydration, occurs frequently in horses with acute colitis and indicates protein loss from the diseased bowel. Hypocalcemia often is observed in horses with hypoalbuminemia and reflects the high proportion of protein-bound calcium in circulation. Ionized (unbound) calcium, which better reflects physiologic calcium homeostasis, usually is normal. Clinicopathologic derangements can vary in severity between cases, depending on the degree of intestinal damage and, in 1 study, severity of electrolyte loss, hemoconcentration, and prerenal azotemia all were predictors of survival.[2]

Measurement of L-lactate concentrations in blood and/or peritoneal fluid has become an increasingly popular diagnostic and prognostic indicator in horses presented for colic and other acute intestinal disorders. Lactate is produced by mammalian cells under anaerobic conditions during global or local tissue ischemia/hypoxia.[3] In horses presented for colic, peritoneal lactate concentrations are higher than blood lactate concentrations (sampled at the same time) in horses with surgical lesions necessitating intestinal resection and anastamosis.[4] In practice, peritoneal fluid lactate concentrations that are twice that of blood are highly suggestive a strangulating surgical lesion. This diagnostic test can be particularly helpful in identifying strangulating lesions early in the course of disease (hours), during which horses may display signs of severe abdominal pain but still have normal hematologic and biochemical profiles.

Blood lactate concentrations alone may also be of prognostic value in horses with acute intestinal disease. In one prospective study evaluating horses presented for surgical colic, higher blood lactate levels at admission and at 24 hours and 72 hours postoperatively was associated with non-survival.[5] Markedly increased blood lactate concentrations at admission are associated with poorer outcomes in horses with large colon volvulus,[6] and horses presenting for colitis with blood lactate concentrations that remain increased in the face of fluid therapy are less likely to survive to discharge.[7,8] In the latter cases, monitoring changes in blood lactate concentration after fluid resuscitation generally is of greater prognostic value than a single measurement.

It has been suggested that hyperlactatemia in horses should be categorized by the physiologic mechanism of excessive lactate production as a means to potentially increase its utility as a diagnostic and prognostic test.[9] Type A hyperlactatemia occurs in response to inadequate tissue perfusion and oxygenation and is observed in horses with dehydration, hypovolemia, and hypoxemia. Type B hyperlactatemia is produced by inflamed and/or ischemic tissues and is observed in horses with inflammatory or strangulating intestinal lesions. Although type A hyperlactatemia generally responds rapidly to restoration of tissue perfusion (often through volume replacement and fluid therapy), type B hyperlactatemia persists until the underlying inflammatory or ischemic condition is corrected. Many horses with inflammatory or ischemic intestinal lesions also are dehydrated and volume-contracted, and increased lactate concentrations in these patients likely represented simultaneous type A and type B hyperlactatemia. Applied clinically, these concepts support serial measurement of blood lactate as a means to identify the source of hyperlactatemia and provide useful information regarding severity and prognosis for survival. This was corroborated by a prospective observational study of horses presenting for gastrointestinal disease, in which a rapid reduction in blood lactate concentration in response to correction of dehydration and restoration of perfusion (type A) was associated with increased survival, whereas persistently increased blood lactate or lactate concentrations that increased in the face of supportive therapy (type B) were associated with more severe intestinal lesions and poorer survival outcomes.[9] This also is true for peritoneal fluid, in which lactate concentrations that remain increased in the face of medical therapy is suggestive of a strangulating or severely inflamed lesion in horses presented for colic.[10]

Lactate concentrations may be measured in blood or peritoneal fluid using either benchtop or portable handheld analyzers, although variable results may be observed with handheld analyzers.[11] The same instrument should be used when comparing blood and peritoneal fluid lactate concentrations in a single patient. Compared with horses, ponies presenting for gastrointestinal disease have higher blood lactate concentrations (median 2.8 mmol/L vs 1.6 mmol/L in 1 study).[12] This difference may be explained by carbohydrate metabolism via the Cori cycle, in which blood glucose (which also was found to be higher in the study ponies) leads to the generation of lactate.[13]

Increased liver enzyme activities occasionally are observed in horses presented for acute gastrointestinal disorders and likely reflect anatomic proximity of the 2 organ systems and direct communication via the biliary system and portal circulation. A retrospective study examining horses with colic observed that increased g-glutamyltransferase (GGT) activity was observed in 49% of horses with right dorsal displacement but only 2% of horses with left dorsal displacement of the large colon, a finding attributed to extrahepatic biliary obstruction from bile duct compression by the displaced colon.[14] Increased liver enzyme activities (GGT, alkaline phosphatase [ALP], and aspartate aminotransferase [AST]) also have been reported in horses with proximal enteritis, which is thought to be due to hepatic injury secondary to ascending enteric bacteria from the common bile duct, absorption of endotoxin from the portal circulation, and/or hepatic hypoxia from systemic inflammation.[15]

Hyperammonemia with clinical signs of encephalopathy occasionally is observed in horses with acute gastrointestinal disease in the absence of concurrent liver disease.[16] These horses present most frequently for diarrhea, colic, and neurologic signs (dullness, blindness, aimless wandering, and obtundation). Blood ammonia concentrations can range from slightly above normal to more than 1000 μmol/L (case 1, discussed later), and higher concentrations at admission were associated with nonsurvival in 1 retrospective report.[16] Hyperammonemia of gastrointestinal origin also has been reported as a cause of neurologic signs and high fatality rates in horses infected with equine coronavirus.[17,18]

Ammonia concentrations in blood samples rapidly increase with storage after collection and, therefore, special handling is required for accurate measurement. Blood should be drawn into EDTA or heparin anticoagulant tubes and centrifuged and plasma separated from red blood cells immediately. If within 1 hour of the laboratory, plasma may be chilled on ice until analysis. If analysis is greater than 1 hour from collection or the sample must be shipped, the separated plasma should be immediately frozen and shipped overnight on ice. It is imperative that the sample remain frozen until analysis, because thawed samples quickly accumulate ammonia.[19]

CHRONIC GASTROINTESTINAL DISEASE

Chronic enteropathies are uncommon in horses and often present clinically as weight loss, diarrhea, and/or recurrent colic. Weight loss is a consistent presenting complaint, reported in 78% of horses in 1 retrospective study.[20] Differential diagnoses for chronic enteropathy include inflammatory bowel disease and alimentary lymphoma, both of which can affect the small intestine, large colon, or both, as well as parasitism, salmonellosis, sand enteropathy, and right dorsal colitis (RDC), which primarily affect the large colon. Although intestinal biopsies (duodenal and/or rectal) can be helpful for determining the nature and extent of intestinal involvement in some horses,[20,21] clinical signs and serum biochemistry results also can provide clues as to the nature and severity of disease. Horses with chronic colonic disease often have impaired water resorption and present with chronic diarrhea. In 1 retrospective study, the clinicopathologic abnormalities detected most frequently in horses with chronic diarrhea included neutrophilia, hypoalbuminemia, hyperglobulinemia, and increased ALP activity.[22] Clinical signs of dehydration and endotoxemia typically observed in acute colitis cases are less common, and many horses with chronic enteropathies are able to compensate for excessive fecal water loss and maintain normal or nearly normal clinicopathologic profiles.

Hypoproteinemia predominantly characterized by hypoalbuminemia is a common finding in horses affected by chronic enteropathy. The severity of hypoproteinemia and hypoalbuminemia may be of prognostic value and was found positively correlated with nonsurvival in a retrospective study examining horses with weight loss despite good appetite.[23] RDC, a complication of nonsteroidal anti-inflammatory drug (NSAID) treatment, is associated with particularly marked protein loss, often resulting in plasma protein concentrations less than 5.0 g/dL and albumin concentrations less than 1.5 g/dL. Although any NSAID is thought to be capable of causing RDC, phenylbutazone, a nonselective cyclooxygenase inhibitor, frequently is implicated. Prolonged administration of phenylbutazone, at 8.8 mg/kg, orally every 24 hours, to 12 healthy adult horses resulted in consistent hypoalbuminemia in 1 clinical trial. Neutropenia also was observed (likely due to marginalization and sequestration in inflamed sections of bowel), and 2 horses developed clinical colitis.[24] The combination of phenylbutazone and flunixin increased the risk for ulcerative damage to the intestinal tract and created severe gastric ulceration and fatal colitis in 1 prospective study.[25] Serial monitoring of albumin concentrations is advisable in horses receiving NSAID administration and a diagnosis of RDC should be strongly considered in horses that develop hypoproteinemia and hypoalbuminemia during treatment. This diagnosis is supported further by observing localized right dorsal colon wall thickening on transabdominal ultrasound (Fig. 1).

In addition to routine hematologic and biochemical testing, the oral glucose absorption test can support a diagnosis of chronic protein-losing enteropathy. This test is simple to perform, requires no specialized equipment, and can be performed

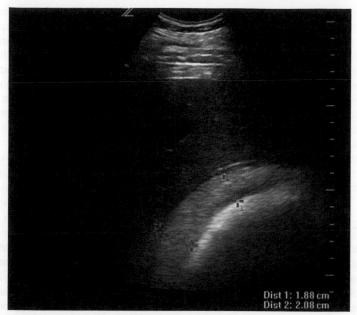

Fig. 1. Ultrasonographic image obtained from the right fourteenth intercostal space of a 3-year-old standardbred gelding with RDC secondary to chronic phenylbutazone administration. The total protein and albumin concentrations were 2.9 g/dL and 0.7 g/dL, respectively, on an initial serum biochemistry panel. The right dorsal colon wall (*blue callipers*) is markedly thickened, measuring between 1.9 cm and 2.1 cm (normal <0.4 cm). The gelding was treated successfully with colloid replacement, misoprostol, gastroprotectants, and discontinuation of the phenylbutazone.

stall-side. In 2 retrospective studies, abnormal glucose absorption was demonstrated in 70% of horses with inflammatory bowel disease[20] and in 57% of horses with chronic diarrhea.[22]

To perform an oral glucose absorption test

1. Fast horse for 12 hours to 18 hours.
2. Measure blood glucose.
3. Administer glucose at 1-g/kg body weight as a 20% solution to the unsedated horse via nasogastric tube.
4. Measure blood glucose every 30 minutes for 2 hours, then every hour for 4 hours.

Accurate serial blood glucose measurements can be obtained easily stall-side using point-of-care glucometers calibrated specifically for horses.[26] In normal horses, blood glucose concentrations should rise to higher than 185% of baseline by 120 minutes post–glucose administration and should return to normal by 6 hours. Horses with malabsorptive enteropathy display a delayed rise in blood glucose and diminished peak concentrations compared with normal horses.[27]

LIVER DISEASE

Liver disease may result from toxic, infectious, hypoxic, neoplastic, vascular, or metabolic causes.[28] Liver disease is detected most commonly by measuring activity of liver-specific enzymes in serum or plasma. Increased hepatic enzyme activity often is a result of secondary liver disease from toxemia, hypoxia, and so forth, and hepatic function remains normal in most horses with these disorders. Primary liver disease most commonly occurs from toxic, infectious, or metabolic causes and may progress to loss of function and clinical signs of hepatic failure. Liver (hepatobiliary) failure occurs when this system has lost some or all of its functionality. Failure generally occurs when greater than 70% of hepatic function is lost and this can be determined by clinical evidence (eg, jaundice, photosensitization, and central nervous system signs) of liver failure, along with abnormal liver function tests, such as bile acids, ammonia, and so forth. It is critical to remember that liver enzyme activities are not indicators of hepatic function! Interpretation of biochemical results is always best made in combination with anamnesis and a thorough clinical examination. Clinical examination, biochemical test results, ultrasonographic findings, and, if indicated, liver biopsy are best used in combination to determine the importance of the liver disease, possible causes, proper treatments, and prognosis.

LIVER ENZYME ACTIVITY IN HORSES WITH PRIMARY LIVER DISEASE

Biochemical testing is imperative when attempting to diagnose liver disease or liver failure. From a clinical perspective, biochemical results can be helpful in narrowing the differential diagnoses for liver analyte changes and, when evaluated over time, help predict prognosis. Biochemical enzyme testing, especially GGT activity, also can be used to identify subclinical hepatotoxin exposure, such as during outbreaks of pyrrolizidine alkaloid toxicity.[29] Enzyme testing can be useful in determining treatment duration, for example, serial GGT measurements to determine duration of antimicrobial treatment of bacterial cholangiohepatitis. Equine liver-specific enzymes include sorbitol dehydrogenase (SDH), glutamate dehydrogenase (GLDH), and GGT, which reflect hepatocellular injury (SDH and GLDH) and cholestasis, biliary necrosis, or hyperplasia (GGT), respectively. AST, lactic dehydrogenase (LDH), and ALP also reflect hepatocellular (AST and LDH) and biliary (ALP) disease, but these enzymes are not liver-specific[28,30,31] (**Table 1**). Increased activities of SDH, GLDH, and AST occur with even mild acute hepatocellular injury, and the magnitude of the enzyme increase may not correspond to the functional status of the liver. SDH is released from the cytosol of the hepatocyte and has a short half-life (approximately 12 hours). Thus, repeated SDH measurements can be helpful in determining resolution or progression of acute hepatocellular disease.[28] The clinical use of SDH measurements for detection of liver disease is affected by its instability in shipped or nonfrozen stored samples. Samples that are refrigerated may be relatively stable for up to 24 hours.[32] GLDH is located in the mitochondria of hepatocytes, and activities are abnormally high in many horses with acute hepatocellular disease. The calculated sensitivities of increased GLDH activity for the detection of hepatic necrosis and of hepatic lipidosis were 78% and 86%, respectively, in 1 study.[31] GLDH is more stable and has a slightly longer half-life than SDH (see **Table 1**). The improved stability of GLDH makes it a recommended test for detecting acute hepatocellular disease when sample shipping is required. Horses with severe chronic fibrosis (cirrhosis) occasionally may have SDH and GLDH activities within normal reference intervals.

GGT is an excellent screening test for hepatic disease in the horse.[33] In the authors' experience, it is rare that a horse with moderate to severe liver disease does not have increased GGT activity. Increases in GGT activity also are highly specific for liver disease because diseases in other body organs (kidney and pancreas) that contain GGT do not result in abnormal serum or plasma GGT activity. GGT activity may continue to increase for several days after an acute hepatic insult has resolved, presumably due to biliary hyperplasia.[28] Although the greatest increase in GGT activity is seen with biliary disease,

Table 1
Serum biochemical enzymes commonly used to detect equine hepatic disease[a]

	Hepatocellular Injury			Biliary Injury/Cholestasis	
	Glutamate Dehydrogenase	Sorbitol Dehydrogenase	Aspartate Aminotransferase	γ-Glutamyltransferase	Alkaline Phosphatase
~Half-life	12–24 h	<12 h	7 d	3 d	3 d
Sensitivity	+++	+++	+++	++++	++
Specificity	+++	++++	+	+++	+
Stability	++	+	++++	++++	++++

+, Lowest; ++++, highest.
[a] These are estimated numbers based on review of available reports.[28,30,31,33,34]

small amounts of GGT can be released after hepatocellular injury.[34] If multiple horses stabled together have increased GGT activity, toxic causes should be considered.

In horses with hepatic disease, relative increases in hepatocellular versus biliary enzyme activities can be helpful when formulating a causative differential diagnostic list. For example, if GGT activity is markedly increased and SDH, GLDH, or AST activities are increased only modestly, diseases that predominantly affect the biliary system, for example, cholangiohepatitis, should be considered most likely. Conversely, if hepatocellular-derived enzyme activity is very high and GGT activity is increased only mildly, then diseases that predominantly affect hepatocytes, for example, serum hepatitis, are more likely.[28] Although somewhat dependent on the duration of disease, many causes of severe liver disease may result in a similar increase in hepatocellular and biliary enzyme activities, for example, pyrrolizidine alkaloid toxicity and hepatic lipidosis.

The magnitude of increase in hepatocellular-derived enzymes may not correspond to hepatic function, and enzyme results should be viewed as a measure of disease and not a measure of function. In addition, the magnitude of changes in hepatocellular enzymes does not determine prognosis. For example, during a 2-year farm investigation of a forage-associated hepatopathy in Europe, more than 70 weanlings, yearlings, and adults had increased GGT (up to 1000 IU/L) and GLDH (up to 1200 IU/L) activities, yet total bilirubin and bile acid concentrations remained within the reference interval in almost all of the horses and no horses demonstrated signs of hepatic failure (Divers TJ 2016, personal observation). Instead, the prognosis for horses with liver disease is best determined by function test abnormalities (discussed later), etiology, fibrosis on liver biopsy, and presence or absence of hepatic encephalopathy.[35]

LIVER ENZYME ACTIVITY IN HORSES WITH SECONDARY LIVER DISEASE

Hepatocellular enzyme activities often are increased with many systemic disorders. This likely reflects inflammatory, vascular, hypoxic, and toxic insults to the liver secondary to the primary disorder and, in these cases, diagnostic and therapeutic attention should focus on the primary disease. Bile acid concentrations, which generally are considered a liver function test, can be increased in some horses with intestinal disorders, such as colic, enteritis, and equine dysautonomia. Moderate to markedly increased bile acid concentrations in horses with colic are associated with a guarded prognosis.[36] Horses with displacement of the left colon to the right occasionally have increases in GGT activity along with increased concentrations of direct (conjugated) bilirubin and bile acids, resulting from obstruction of bile flow.[14] These horses have an excellent prognosis after correction of the displacement.

A small number of racehorses may have moderate increases in GGT (50–140 IU/L) activity with either no or only mild increases in other liver-derived enzyme activity, including ALP. The serum/plasma GGT activity generally remains in the 50-IU/L to 140-IU/L range for weeks in these horses if kept in work. Studies have demonstrated that GGT activity is correlated to cumulative training load and racing frequency and considered a maladaptation to training.[37–40] Oxidative stress has been hypothesized as a cause.[28] The incidence of this increased GGT activity in racehorses in 1 study was 18%,[41] but in some stables it may be higher. This abnormality has not been proved to affect performance, although many trainers believe there is a correlation between the high GGT syndrome and reduced performance.

LIVER FUNCTION TESTS

Liver function tests become abnormal only after 70% or more of hepatic function is lost.[42] Liver function test include increased direct (conjugated) and indirect (unconjugated) bilirubin concentrations, ammonia and bile acid concentrations, and coagulation tests, such as the prothrombin and activated partial thromboplastin times.[28,42,43] In the authors' experience, an increase in conjugated bilirubin above the normal upper limit of the reference interval is a common finding in horses with liver failure. When the abnormally high conjugated bilirubin concentration comprises 25% or more of the total bilirubin concentration, this is suggestive of a predominant biliary and obstructive disease.[44] Increases in conjugated bilirubin (which is water-soluble) result in bilirubinuria, which may be detected by urine test strips or observing green-colored bubbles after shaking the urine. Rarely, a horse without liver disease has a positive bilirubin reading on the urine test strip. Increased unconjugated bilirubin concentration is a moderately sensitive test for liver failure but lacks specificity because increases also may occur with anorexia and hemolysis or, on rare occasions, may be seen in a healthy horse.[31] The latter condition may be caused by a congenital deficiency in glucuronyl transferase, and affected horses can maintain total bilirubin concentrations of 9 mg/dL or greater.[45]

Bile acid concentrations above 20 μmol/L are a good predictor of liver failure.[33,35] Milder increases (up to 20 μmol/L) may occur in a few horses without hepatic disease that are anorexic for 2 or more days.[46] Horses with chronic liver disease and persistently increased bile acid concentrations greater than 20 μmol/L have a guarded to poor prognosis.[35,47] Bile acid concentrations should not be used as a predictor of prognosis in horses with acute liver disease.

In states of negative energy balance, triglyceride concentrations frequently are increased in horses but hepatic lipidosis resulting in liver failure rarely occurs unless visible lipemia is noted.[48] Therefore, high triglyceride concentrations alone should not be used to diagnose hepatic lipidosis and liver failure.

Albumin concentrations rarely are low in horses with acute (6%) or chronic (18%) liver failure, and hypoalbuminemia is neither a sensitive nor specific test for liver failure in the horse.[49] Conversely, globulins are increased in 48% of horses with liver failure.[49] The albumin-to-globulin ratio is more likely to be low in horses with chronic versus acute liver disease and failure.[49] Although an inconsistent finding, urea nitrogen concentrations may be low with liver failure, presumably due to decreased synthesis in the urea cycle.[50]

Clotting times often are increased in horses with liver failure due to insufficient hepatic synthesis of clotting factors II, V, VII, IX, X, XI, and XII.[51] Coagulation abnormalities may not be detected in some horses with liver failure, even in those with obstructive biliary disease and failure.[44] This is somewhat surprising considering the importance of bile acids in the absorption of vitamin K and the importance of vitamin K in synthesis of activated coagulation factors II, VII, IX, and X, along with the inhibitors proteins C and S.[44] Regardless, clinical bleeding is uncommon and liver biopsies can be performed safely in most cases.[51] One explanation for the safety of liver biopsy in horses with fulminant hepatic disease could be that platelet counts often remain within reference intervals in most horses with liver failure. Fibrinogen, an acute-phase protein made in the liver, usually is normal or mildly decreased in horses with acute or chronic liver failure, except in horses with cholangiohepatitis, where it may be high secondary to inflammation.[44]

OTHER CLINICOPATHOLOGIC ABNORMALITIES IN LIVER DISEASE

Lactate concentrations frequently are high and bicarbonate concentrations are usually low in horses with fulminant hepatic failure.[28] The high lactate concentration likely is due to a combination of decreased hepatic clearance and increased production from hemodynamic alterations found with hepatic failure and likely responsible for the low bicarbonate concentration. Glucose concentrations often are surprisingly normal in most adult horses with hepatic failure but, in some cases, glucose may be very low.[52,53] Hematocrit, iron concentrations, and percentage iron saturation occasionally are high in horses with severe liver disease, in particular those with acute necrosis. The erythrocytosis can persist despite adequate rehydration. These clinicopathologic findings should not be interpreted as iron toxicity because that diagnosis can be confirmed only by histologic evidence of hemochromatosis.

CASE 1

A 19-year-old Appaloosa gelding was examined because of an acute onset of diarrhea and fever. Heart rate was 56 beats per minute, mucous membranes were abnormally red, and capillary refill time was 5 seconds. Blood samples were submitted for hemogram, biochemical profile, lactate concentration, and blood polymerase chain reaction (PCR) testing for *Neorickettsia risticii,* along with fecal testing for other common enteric infectious agents. Initial treatment included intravenously administered crystalloids and oxytetracycline. Supportive treatment with misoprostol and di-tri-octahedral smectite (Bio-Sponge Platinum Performance, Buellton Calif. USA) administered orally and flunixin meglumine administered intravenously, and distal limb cryotherapy occurred within 1 hour of hospital admission. The horse had a good clinical response to treatment over the first 18 hours but on day 2 developed acute neurologic signs, which included circling, head pressing, and ataxia. The ammonia concentration was markedly increased (**Table 2**) and treatment with orally administered lactulose and intravenously administered mannitol was initiated. Commercial equine plasma and a synthetic colloid also were administered intravenously on days 3 and 4, respectively. The blood PCR for *N risticii* was positive. The horse made a full recovery and was discharged from the hospital after 5 days.

Case Discussion

Hyperammonemia may develop in a small number of horses with acute gastrointestinal disease. The magnitude of the hyperammonemia is somewhat unique to the horse and may be related to microbiome changes in the gut (increased amounts of ammonia-producing bacteria) and/or increased intestinal permeability. In these cases, neurologic signs develop quickly and may lead to death in less than 24 hours, although some horses may have a rapid (<48 hours) decrease in ammonia concentrations and complete recovery if the primary intestinal disease resolves. The authors are not aware of a horse with ammonia concentrations this high that survived.

Interpretation of clinical pathologic data

- HCT of 66%, due to hypovolemia from gastrointestinal fluid losses (dehydration)
- Inflammatory leukogram: the most common leukogram findings in acute severe colitis is leukopenia, due to a neutropenia with a left shift and concurrent toxic change in neutrophils. Not all horses have neutropenia, as observed in this case. A mild monocytosis is a commonly observed feature of *N risticii* infection in horses.
- Lower than expected total protein (especially albumin) concentration considering the relative erythrocytosis and estimated degree of dehydration. This combination occurs frequently in horses with acute colitis and indicates protein loss from the diseased bowel. The marked decrease in total protein and albumin concentrations between days 1 and 3 also is common in horses with colitis due to

Table 2
Pertinent clinical pathologic findings for case 1

	Day 1	Day 3	Reference Interval
HCT	66	41	34%–46%
White blood cell count	12.2	6.3	5.2–10.1 thou/μL
Neutrophils	4.4	3.3	2.7–6.6 thou/μL
Band neutrophils	3.2	0	0.0–0.1 thou/μL
Monocytes	1.8	0.8	0.0–0.6 thou/μL
Platelets	Adequate[a]	Adequate[a]	94–232 thou/μL
Sodium	115	132	134–142 mEq/L
Potassium	3.2	3.2	2.4–4.8 mEq/L
Chloride	69	106	95–104 mEq/L
Bicarbonate	9	19	24–31 mEq/L
UN	84	24	10–22 mg/dL
Creatinine	5.5	1.4	0.8–1.5 mg/dL
Total protein	6.3	3.0	5.4–7.0 g/dL
Albumin	2.3	1.5	2.9–3.6 g/dL
L-Lactate	9.16	1.6	<1.5 mmol/L
Ammonia	1495 (day 2)	695 23 (day 4)	<150 μg/dL

[a] Platelet clumping noted on smear precluded quantification.

ongoing protein-losing enteropathy. The resultant decrease in colloid osmotic pressure can make crystalloid therapy less effective in maintaining intravascular volume because the administered crystalloid fluids tend to shift more rapidly out of the intravascular space.

- Severe prerenal azotemia, which largely resolved with appropriate fluid therapy.
- Hyponatremia and hypochloremia are both common findings with acute colitis in horses. In this horse, the measured decrease in the negatively charged ions, chloride (change of −31 mEq/L) and albumin (−0.6 g/dL or −2.0 mEq/L)[a], were greater than the decrease in the positively charged sodium (change of −23 mEq/L)[a], indicating that other negatively charged ions are likely increased. In this horse, the bicarbonate concentration was also very low (change of −18 mEq/L)[a] and L-lactate concentration was very high, indicating a metabolic acidosis due to L-lactate. Other unmeasured anions, such as D-lactate or acids accumulating from the severe prerenal azotemia, also may have been present to help explain both the strong ion difference and the metabolic acidosis.
- Hyperlactemia often is present in horses with acute severe colitis as a result of hypovolemia and endotoxin/cytokine effects on global tissue perfusion (type A) with additional lactate production from the local damage to the bowel wall (type B). This horse had an excellent initial response to treatment and lactate concentrations decreased quickly following fluid therapy. Horses that do not have substantial decreases in lactate concentrations after fluid resuscitation have a more guarded prognosis.[8,9]

[a] Changes in ions calculated by subtracting patient value from mid normal range value.

CASE 2

A 5-year-old previously healthy miniature horse mare presented with acute depression, icterus, anorexia, and inability to open the jaw. The mare was diagnosed with selenium-deficient masseter myopathy with secondary negative energy balance and hepatic lipidosis. Blood analysis included hemogram, biochemical profile, and lactate concentrations (**Table 3**). A free-catch urine sample was dark brown, with a USG of 1.025, and a urine dipstick test revealed bilirubinuria and positive heme (blood) reaction. The mare was treated with intramuscular and oral selenium and vitamin E and supported with partial parenteral nutrition and made a full recovery. The prognosis for hepatic lipidosis can be excellent regardless of the triglyceride concentration if the triggering disease is resolved promptly and proper nutritional support is provided.

Interpretation of Laboratory Findings

- Liver disease and failure: this mare has evidence of liver disease (increased hepatocellular and biliary enzyme activities) in addition to muscle disease (increased creatine kinase [CK] activity). The increase in total and direct bilirubin concentration along with the clinical signs and other biochemical findings support a diagnosis of liver dysfunction (failure). The increased AST activity was a result of both muscle and liver disease.
  - The marked increase in SDH (>30 times the upper reference limit) and milder increase in GGT (slightly >3 times the upper reference limit) with 11% of the total bilirubin being direct bilirubin suggest that hepatocellular injury is more severe than cholestasis.
  - The normal SDH activity on day 5 reflects both the rapid improvement in the disease and the short half-life of SDH. GGT activity is still increased on day 5 due to the longer half-life of GGT and likely from some continued biliary proliferation.
- Rhabdomyolysis: increased muscle enzyme activities (CK and AST) and positive heme reaction on urine dipstick due to myoglobin, all of which improved during hospitalization. The greater decrease in CK activity during 5 days of hospitalization is due to the shorter half-life (hours) compared with AST (days).

Table 3
Pertinent clinical pathologic findings for case 2

	Day 1	Day 3	Day 5	Reference Interval
Packed cell volume	43	42	42	34%–46%
Total solids (by refractometer)	7.2	6.9	6.8	5.2–7.8 g/dL
pH (venous)	7.29	7.35	—	7.32–7.43
Bicarbonate	20	26	26	25–32 mEq/L
L-Lactate	3.5	1.8	—	0.8–1.8 mmol/L
Creatinine	2.2	1.6	1.5	0.8–2.0 mg/dL
CK	57,040	21,984	1142	142–548 U/L
AST	13,030	10,780	4474	199–374 U/L
SDH	362	118	5	0–11 U/L
GGT	77	146	103	8–29 U/L
Total bilirubin	6.2	2.6	1.9	0.5–2.1 mg/dL
Direct bilirubin	0.7	0.3	0.2	0.1–0.3 mg/dL
Triglycerides	1929	75	27	14–65 mg/dL

- Negative energy balance with hypertriglyceridemia: miniature horses are at increased risk for developing hypertriglyceridemia, hyperlipemia, and hepatic lipidosis in response to anorexia. The increase in circulating lipids reflects increased mobilization of fat stores as well as decreased clearance/metabolism of lipids by the liver. Treatment with intravenous dextrose, parenteral nutrition, and/or enteral nutrition often results in rapid reduction in triglyceride concentrations and resolution of hepatic lipidosis.
- The acidemia with a metabolic acidosis (low venous pH and low bicarbonate), mildly increased creatinine concentration (likely prerenal azotemia), and abnormally high L-lactate concentration are likely a result of dehydration and diminished tissue perfusion, although some of the increase in L-lactate may have occurred because of decreased hepatic dysfunction/metabolism. Dehydration is further supported by the USG of 1.025. Venous pH and creatinine and lactate concentrations all normalized rapidly in response to intravenous crystalloid fluid therapy.

DISCLOSURE

The authors have nothing to disclose.

REFERENCES

1. Gomez DE, Arroyo LG, Stampfli HR, et al. Physiochemical interpretation of acid-base abnormalities in 54 adult horses with acute severe colitis and diarrhea. J Vet Intern Med 2013;27(3):548–53.
2. Bertin FR, Reising A, Slovis NM, et al. Clinical and clinicopathological factors associated with survival in 44 horses with equine neorickettsiosis (Potomac Horse Fever). J Vet Intern Med 2013;27(6):1528–34.
3. Latson KM, Nieto JE, Beldomenico PM, et al. Evaluation of peritoneal fluid lactate as a marker of intestinal ischaemia in equine colic. Equine Vet J 2005;37(4): 342–6.
4. Pye J, Espinosa-Mur P, Roca R, et al. Preoperative factors associated with resection and anastomosis in horses presenting with strangulating lesions of the small intestine. Vet Surg 2019. https://doi.org/10.1111/vsu.13184.
5. Radcliffe RM, Divers TJ, Fletcher DJ, et al. Evaluation of L-lactate and cardiac troponin I in horses undergoing emergency abdominal surgery. J Vet Emerg Crit Care 2012;22(3):313–9.
6. Johnston K, Holcombe SJ, Hauptman JG. Plasma lactate as a predictor of colonic viability and survival after 360 degrees volvulus of the ascending colon in horses. Vet Surg 2007;36(6):563–7.
7. Hashimoto-Hill S, Magdesian KG, Kass PH. Serial measurement of lactate concentration in horses with acute colitis. J Vet Intern Med 2011;25(6):1414–9.
8. Peterson MB, Tolver A, Husted L, et al. Repeated measurements of blood lactate concentration as a prognostic indicator marker in horses with acute colitis evaluated with classification and regression trees (CART) and random forest analysis. Vet J 2016;213:18–23.
9. Tennent-Brown BS, Wilkins PA, Lindborg S, et al. Sequential plasma lactate concentrations as prognostic indicators in adult equine emergencies. J Vet Intern Med 2010;24:198–205.
10. Peloso JG, Cohen ND. Use of serial measurements of peritoneal fluid lactate concentration to identify strangulating intestinal lesions in referred horses with signs of colic. J Am Vet Med Assoc 2012;240(10):1208–17.

11. Nieto JE, Dechant JE, le Jeune SS, et al. Evaluation of 3 handheld portable analyzers for measurement of L-lactate concentrations in blood and peritoneal fluid of horses with colic. Vet Surg 2015;44(3):366–72.

12. Dunkel B, Kapff JE, Naylor RJ, et al. Blood lactate concentrations in ponies and miniature horses with gastrointestinal disease. Equine Vet J 2013;45(6):666–70.

13. Dunkel B, Mason CJ, Chang YM. Retrospective evaluation of the association between admission blood glucose and l-lactate concentrations in ponies and horses with gastrointestinal disease (2008-2016): 545 cases. J Vet Emerg Crit Care 2019. https://doi.org/10.1111/vec.12851.

14. Gardner RB, Nydam DV, Mohammed HO, et al. Serum gamma glutamyl transferase activity in horses with right or left displacements of the large colon. J Vet Intern Med 2005;19(5):761–4.

15. Davis JL, Blikslager AT, Catto K, et al. A retrospective analysis of hepatic injury in horses with proximal enteritis (1984-2002). J Vet Intern Med 2003;17(6):896–901.

16. Dunkel B, Chaney KP, Dallap-Schaer BL, et al. Putative intestinal hyperammonemia in horses: 36 cases. Equine Vet J 2011;43(2):133–40.

17. Fielding CL, Higgins JK, Higgins JC, et al. Disease associated with equine coronavirus infection and high case fatality rate. J Vet Intern Med 2015;29(1):307–10.

18. Giannitti F, Diab S, Mete A, et al. Necrotizing enteritis and hyperammonemic encephalopathy associated with equine coronavirus infection in equids. Vet Pathol 2015;52(6):1148–56.

19. Lindner A, Bauer S. Effect of temperature, duration of storage and sampling procedure on ammonia concentration in equine blood plasma. Eur J Clin Chem Clin Biochem 1993;31(7):473–6.

20. Boshuizen B, Ploeg M, Dewulf J, et al. Inflammatory bowel disease (IBD) in horses: a retrospective study exploring the value of different diagnostic approaches. BMC Vet Res 2018;14(1):21.

21. Divers TJ, Pelligrini-Masini A, McDonough S. Diagnosis of inflammatory bowel disease in a Hackney pony by gastroduodenal endoscopy and biopsy and successful treatment with corticosteroids. Equine Vet Educ 2006;18(6):284–7.

22. Love S, Mair TS, Hillyer MH. Chronic diarrhea in adult horses: a review of 51 cases. Vet Rec 1992;130(11):217–9.

23. Metcalfe LV, More SJ, Duggan V, et al. A retrospective study of horses investigated for weight loss despite a good appetite (2002-2011). Equine Vet J 2013; 45(3):340–5.

24. McConnico RS, Morgan TW, Williams CC, et al. Pathophysiologic effects of phenylbutazone on the right dorsal colon in horses. Am J Vet Res 2008;69(11): 1496–505.

25. Reed SK, Messer NT, Tessman RK, et al. Effect of phenylbutazone alone or in combination with flunixin meglumine on blood protein concentrations in horses. Am J Vet Res 2006;67(3):398–402.

26. Hackett ES, McCue PM. Evaluation of a veterinary glucometer for use in horses. J Vet Intern Med 2010;24(3):617–21.

27. Murphy D, Reid SWJ, Love S. Modified oral glucose tolerance test as an indicator of small intestinal pathology in horses. Vet Rec 1997;140:342–3.

28. Divers TJ. The equine liver in health and disease. Proceeding of the American Proc Am Assoc Equine Practit 2015;6:66–103.

29. Curran JM, Sutherland RJ, Peet RL. A screening test for subclinical liver disease in horses affected by pyrrolizidine alkaloid toxicosis. Aust Vet J 1996;74:236–40.

30. Bernard WV, Divers TJ. Variations in serum sorbitol dehydrogenase, aspartate transaminase, and isoenzyme 5 of lactate dehydrogenase activities in horses given carbon tetrachloride. Am J Vet Res 1989;50(5):622–3.
31. West HJ. Clinical and pathological studies in horses with hepatic disease. Equine Vet J 1996;28:146–56.
32. Horney BS, Honor DJ, MacKenzie A, et al. Stability of sorbitol dehydrogenase activity in bovine and equine sera. Vet Clin Pathol 1993;22:5–9.
33. McGorum BC, Murphy D, Love S, et al. Clinicopathological features of equine primary hepatic disease: a review of 50 cases. Vet Rec 1999;145:134–9.
34. Noonan NE. Variations of plasma enzymes in the pony and the dog after carbon tetrachloride administration. Am J Vet Res 1981;42(4):674–8.
35. Durham AE, Newton JR, Smith KC, et al. Retrospective analysis of historical, clinical, ultrasonographic, serum biochemical and haematological data in prognostic evaluation of equine liver disease. Equine Vet J 2003;35:542–7.
36. Underwood C, Southwood LL, Walton RM, et al. Hepatic and metabolic changes in surgical colic patients: a pilot study. J Vet Emerg Crit Care 2010;20(6):578–86.
37. Snow DH, Harris P. Enzymes as markers of physical fitness and training of racing horses. Adv Clin Enzymol 1988;6:251–8.
38. McGowan C. Clinical pathology in the racing horse: the role of clinical pathology in assessing fitness and performance in the racehorse. Vet Clin North Am Equine Pract 2008;24:405–22.
39. Mack SJ, Kirkby K, Malalana F, et al. Elevations in serum muscle enzyme activities in racehorses due to unaccustomed exercise and training. Vet Rec 2014; 174:145.
40. Leleu C, Haentjens F. Morphological, haemato-biochemical and endocrine changes in young Standardbreds with 'maladaptation' to early training. Equine Vet J Suppl 2010;38:171–8.
41. Ramsay JD, Evanoff R, Mealey RH, et al. The prevalence of elevated gamma-glutamyltransferase and sorbitol dehydrogenase activity in racing Thoroughbreds and their associations with viral infection. Equine Vet J 2019;51(6):738–42.
42. Schendl MJ, Redhead DN, Fearon KCH. The value of residual liver volume as a predictor of hepatic dysfunction and infection after major liver resection. Gut 2005;54(2):289–96.
43. Durham AE. Hepatitis in horses. In: Weber O, Protzer U, editors. Comparative hepatitis. Basel (Switzerland): Birkhauser Verlag; 2008. p. 245–64.
44. Peek SF, Divers TJ. Medical treatment of cholangiohepatitis and cholelithiasis in mature horses: 9 cases (1991-1998). Equine Vet J 2000;32:301–6.
45. Divers TJ, Schappel KA, Sweeney RW, et al. Persistent hyperbilirubinemia in a healthy thoroughbred horse. Cornell Vet 1993;83(3):237–42.
46. Hoffmann WE, Baker G, Rieser S, et al. Alterations in selected serum biochemical constituents in equids after induced hepatic disease. Am J Vet Res 1987;48: 1343–7.
47. Dunkel B, Jones SA, Pinilla MJ, et al. Serum bile acid concentrations, histopathological features, and short-, and long-term survival in horses with hepatic disease. J Vet Intern Med 2015;29(2):644–50.
48. Dunkel B, McKenzie HC 3rd. Severe hypertriglyceridaemia in clinically ill horses: diagnosis, treatment and outcome. Equine Vet J 2003;35:590–5.
49. Parraga ME, Carlson GP, Thurmond M. Serum protein concentrations in horses with severe liver disease: a retrospective study and review of the literature. J Vet Intern Med 1995;9:154–61.

50. Tennant BC. Hepatic function. In: Kaneko JJ, Harvey JW, Bruss ML, editors. Clinical biochemistry of domestic animals. 6th edition. Maryland Heights (MO): Elsevier Academic Press; 1997. p. 379–413.

51. Johns IC, Sweeney RW. Coagulation abnormalities and complications after percutaneous liver biopsy in horses. J Vet Intern Med 2008;22:185–9.

52. Tomlinson JE, Kapoor A, Kumar A, et al. Viral testing of 18 consecutive cases of equine serum hepatitis: a prospective study (2014-2018). J Vet Intern Med 2019; 33(1):251–7.

53. Aleman M, Costa LRR, Crowe C, et al. Presumed neuroglycopenia caused by severe hypoglycemia in horses. Vet Intern Med 2018;32(5):1731–9.

The Sick Adult Horse
Renal Clinical Pathologic Testing and Urinalysis

Harold C. Schott II, DVM, PhD*, Melissa M. Esser, DVM, MS

KEYWORDS

- Azotemia • Acute kidney injury • Chronic kidney disease • Urine-specific gravity
- Enzymuria • Symmetric dimethylarginine • Furosemide

KEY POINTS

- Clinicopathologic evaluation of kidney disease includes measures of renal function (glomerular filtration rate, tubular modification of filtrate) and biomarkers of renal injury.
- Acute kidney injury (AKI) is usually a secondary disease process and increases morbidity, length of hospital stay, and mortality of the primary disorder. Early AKI identification is essential for initiating therapies aimed at minimizing renal damage and improving outcome.
- Early recognition of chronic kidney disease is important to allow interventions that may slow progression and prolong life for affected equids.
- Examination findings (eg, urine production) and clinicopathologic testing (eg, serum biochemistry, urinalysis) remain useful in assessing renal status in sick adult horses.

TERMINOLOGY FOR ALTERATIONS IN KIDNEY FUNCTION AND KIDNEY INJURY

The terminology applied to renal dysfunction or injury has changed. Use of the term *prerenal failure* to describe acute, reversible decreases in renal blood flow (RBF), glomerular filtration rate (GFR), and urine output (UO), that may or may not progress to clinical renal failure, has fallen out of favor because the term was not well defined and "reversible" changes in renal function were associated with increased mortality.[1] Consequently, the term *acute kidney injury* (AKI) was introduced to increase awareness of renal injury (subclinical and clinical) that accompanies sudden decreases in RBF, GFR, and UO. Over the past 15 years, the definition of AKI has evolved from the RIFLE (*Risk-Injury-Failure-Loss-End-stage*, introduced in 2004)[2] and *Acute Kidney Injury Network* (AKIN, introduced in 2007)[3] staging systems to the *Kidney Disease: Improving Global Outcomes (KDIGO) Clinical Practice Guideline for Acute Kidney Injury* staging system in 2012.[4] In all 3 systems, the magnitude of increase in serum

Department of Large Animal Clinical Sciences, Veterinary Medical Center, College of Veterinary Medicine, Michigan State University, Room D-202, 736 Wilson Road, East Lansing, MI 48824, USA
* Corresponding author.
E-mail address: schott@msu.edu

Vet Clin Equine 36 (2020) 121–134
https://doi.org/10.1016/j.cveq.2019.12.003
0749-0739/20/© 2019 Elsevier Inc. All rights reserved.

creatinine (Cr) concentration within 48 hours to 7 days is combined with duration and severity of oliguria to categorize AKI from stage 1 to stage 3. Furthermore, KDIGO guidelines provided consensus recommendations for prevention/limitation of AKI in at-risk patients and a conceptual model for AKI, emphasizing that both decreased GFR and direct injury to renal cells combine to incite AKI (**Fig. 1**).[4] Another consensus statement from 2017 further refined AKI to separate reversible AKI (Cr returning to baseline within 48 hours) from persisting AKI.[5] This group also proposed that *acute kidney disease* (AKD) be defined as azotemia persisting for 7 to 90 days after onset of renal injury. When azotemia persists after 90 days, the term *chronic kidney disease* (CKD) is used. This recent statement emphasized that the intermediate phase of AKD is least understood and provided examples of courses of recovery or disease progression.[5] Using any of these classification systems, AKI has been documented in 7% to 18% of hospitalized human patients, and approximately 50% of patients admitted to intensive care units.[6] Furthermore, AKI is nearly always a secondary complication in patients with sepsis or cardiac disease, or receiving intravenous contrast agents and concurrent AKI increases patient morbidity and duration of hospitalization. Unfortunately, mortalities with more severe AKI (AKIN or KDIGO stages 2 or 3) in hospitalized patients remain high (~50%) and have declined little over the past 20 years.[7,8] Thus, early recognition of AKI and interventions to limit progression and reverse kidney damage are much needed.

ACUTE KIDNEY INJURY AND CHRONIC KIDNEY DISEASE IN EQUIDS

Less data exist to document the prevalence of AKI, AKD, CKD, and outcomes in horses. In the authors' hospital, mild azotemia (arbitrarily defined as Cr >2.5 mg/dL at

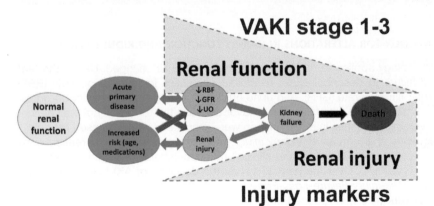

Fig. 1. Conceptual model for AKI: Blue circles represent risk factors for development of AKI, whereas green circles are the 2 primary contributors to AKI; gray triangles indicate the degree of change over time in function and injury, as characterized by the VAKI stage and magnitude of increase in serum and/or urine biomarkers of renal injury. Outcomes can be reversible renal failure or death. FCINa, fractional sodium clearance; GGT/Cr, ratio of urine gamma glutamyl transferase activity to urine creatinine concentration. (*Adapted from* McCullough PA, Kellum JA, Mehta RL, et al. Kidney Disease: Improving Global Outcomes (KDIGO) Acute Kidney Injury Work Group. KDIGO Clinical Practice Guideline for Acute Kidney Injury. Kidney Int, Suppl 2012;2:1-138; with permission.)

admission) was detected in ~20% of horses in 1997 and 2000,[9] translating to an annual incidence of ~5% of the total equine caseload (chemistry profiles were performed in ~20% of cases). As in human patients, AKI was almost always a secondary complication of another disease, usually gastrointestinal (GI) disorders. Horses with moderate azotemia (arbitrarily defined as Cr of 5–10 mg/dL at admission, <1% of caseload) had a mortality of 30% to 45%. However, mortality was 100% for patients with severe azotemia (arbitrarily defined as Cr >10 mg/dL), with the exception of neonates with spurious hypercreatininemia.[10] In another study of 79 horses with GI disease, in which at least 2 Cr measurements were performed 72 hours apart, horses with persisting azotemia (26/79, 33%) were 3 times more likely to die or be euthanized (42% mortality) than horses in which Cr normalized.[11] Recently, the Veterinary Acute Kidney Injury (VAKI) staging system (**Table 1**), initially adapted for dogs[12] from the KDIGO classification, was used to determine prevalence of AKI in hospitalized horses with at least 2 serum Cr measurements (between 24 hours and 7 days of hospitalization).[13] Of 325 cases (mostly GI emergencies), 4.3% (n = 14) had baseline azotemia (mean Cr 2.4 mg/dL, range 1.9–3.5 mg/dL), which normalized during hospitalization, whereas 14.7% (n = 48) developed AKI (44 VAKI stage 1 and 4 VAKI stage 2) during hospitalization. Mortalities were 29% for horses with baseline azotemia versus 12% for horses developing reversible AKI during hospitalization. During the same time period, 3 horses (<1% of caseload) were admitted for evaluation of renal disease, supporting a low prevalence of primary renal disease (usually CKD). For future investigation of AKI in horses, the timeframe for changes in Cr for AKI staging should be clearly defined (eg, 48 hours to 7 days).

Limited data support a 0.1% to 0.2% prevalence of CKD in horses, which increases to 0.5% in horses older than 15 years of age.[14] These data likely underestimate CKD prevalence because clinicopathologic testing is not routinely performed in healthy older horses. The International Renal Interest Society (IRIS) has developed a CKD staging system to identify dogs and cats in earlier stages of CKD when interventions may be more effective in slowing progression.[15] A similar staging system has not been developed for horses. Unfortunately, many horses have advanced disease (IRIS stage 4 with serum Cr >5.0 mg/dL) when CKD is initially recognized.

ASSESSMENT FOR RENAL DISEASE IN SICK ADULT HORSES

When evaluating adult horses with various medical and surgical disorders, renal function should be considered. Early AKI detection should limit morbidity and improve

Table 1		
Proposed veterinary acute kidney injury scoring system for horses, using an increase in serum creatinine concentration from admission value (or baseline value if available) during the initial 7 days of disease process		
VAKI Stage	**Change in sCr from Baseline**	
Stage 0	Increase in sCr <150% from baseline	
Stage 1	Increase in sCr of 150%–199% or an absolute increase of ≥0.3 mg/dL (≥26.5 μmol/L) from baseline	
Stage 2	Increase in sCr of 200%–299% from baseline	
Stage 3	Increase in sCr of ≥300% from baseline or an absolute increase to ≥4.0 mg/dL (≥354 μmol/L)	

From Savage VL, Marr CM, Bailey M, et al. Prevalence of acute kidney injury in a population of hospitalized horses. J Vet Intern Med 2019;330:2294-301; with permission.

outcome in patients with secondary renal disease. If dehydration or compromised hemodynamic status is present, the expected physiologic response would be acute reductions in RBF, GFR, and UO. As an example, when healthy horses were deprived of water for 3 days, UO decreased to 1.25 to 2.5 mL/min (0.15–0.30 mL/kg/h); urine-specific gravity (USG) increased to 1.040 to 1.050, and urine osmolality increased to 1500 to 2000 mOsm/kg during the second and third days of water deprivation.[16] Of interest, UO in these dehydrated horses was less that the accepted definition for oliguria in humans (UO <0.5 mL/kg/h for 6–12 hours or UO <0.3 mL/kg/h for 24 hours).[5] Finally, a complete history can provide clues as to the duration of decreased renal perfusion and use of potentially nephrotoxic medications. Questioning owners about long-standing excessive drinking and urination habits may provide evidence for pre-existing CKD, especially for patients with weight loss. With hospitalization, observation for urination (and sample collection) when a horse is initially moved into a stall should be considered an essential component of physical examination. Even dehydrated horses may void a small amount of urine when placed into a stall with fresh bedding. Although often overlooked, collection of the first urine sample can provide valuable information and should be done before treatment, because α_2-agonists or fluid therapy can artifactually decrease urine tonicity.[17,18] Although not ideal, urine can also be collected from the floor. If urine is not voided spontaneously, a simple collection device can be suspended below the prepuce (**Fig. 2**) or a bladder catheter can be passed in mares to collect an initial sample.

CLINICOPATHOLOGIC ASSESSMENT FOR RENAL DISEASE

Clinicopathologic testing of kidney function and damage in sick adult horses includes assessment for azotemia, anemia, and inflammation; measurement of blood and urine electrolyte concentrations; urinalysis; and measurement of other urine biomarkers of renal injury.[19,20] When azotemia is detected, the initial step is to determine whether the patient has AKI, CKD, or an acute exacerbation of CKD ("acute-on-chronic" disease). Unfortunately, iatrogenic, drug-associated nephrotoxicity remains an important contributor to AKI in horses.

Estimates of Glomerular Filtration Rate

Serum/plasma urea nitrogen (UN) and Cr concentrations, as indirect estimates of GFR, are traditionally used to assess renal function. Unfortunately, neither are

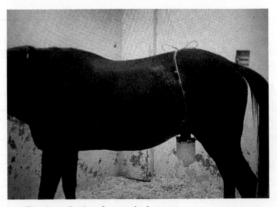

Fig. 2. Simple urine collection device for male horses.

sensitive indicators of decreased renal function because values typically do not increase above upper reference interval limits until GFR is reduced by $\geq 75\%$. However, once above the reference interval, small increases become sensitive indicators of further GFR deterioration, with doubling of values indicating a 50% decline in renal function. Because Cr is released as a degradation product of skeletal muscle creatine, breed and sex differences in muscle mass may affect concentrations, as documented in dogs.[21] The commonly used Jaffe reaction also measures non-Cr chromogens that may account for 45% to 50% of the Cr concentration in dogs.[21] Finally, a small amount of Cr can be eliminated by tubular secretion; thus, Cr can overestimate GFR.

The UN:Cr ratio can also be used in sick horses. In hypovolemic horses with acute medical and surgical problems, clinical experience finds that Cr increases more rapidly than UN, leading to a UN:Cr ratio less than 10:1. A greater increase in Cr than UN is speculated to be due to greater diffusibility of UN versus Cr. In contrast, with CKD, the UN:Cr ratio often exceeds 10:1 and may exceed 15:1.[22] Because a sudden decrease in RBF and GFR typically leads to greater increases in Cr than UN, Cr is the best test to identify acute changes in renal function over short durations in sick horses. With CKD, the UN:Cr ratio may also be useful in assessing dietary protein intake because values greater than 15:1 may suggest excessive dietary protein intake, and increased urea production, or upper GI bleeding.[22]

Novel Biomarkers of Glomerular Filtration Rate

To better estimate GFR, novel serum biomarkers have been investigated in horses, including cystatin C (CysC) and symmetric dimethylarginine (SDMA). CysC is a small (13 kDa) cysteine protease inhibitor released by all cells at a fairly constant rate. It is almost exclusively eliminated by glomerular filtration.[23,24] Thus, as GFR and glomerular filtration of CysC decreases, serum CysC concentration increases. Essentially all CysC is reabsorbed in the proximal tubule, with scant CysC in urine.[23] Increases in serum CysC, and increased urinary CysC excretion, appear to be sensitive indicators of AKI in human patients, but may not be superior to Cr.[25-27] However, serum CysC yields lower GFR estimates than Cr in CKD, allowing earlier intervention to slow disease progression.[24,28] Measurement of CysC has been assessed in dogs and cats,[24] but initial attempts to measure CysC in equine plasma with a human-based immunoassay were unsuccessful.[29]

Measurement of SDMA concentration to estimate GFR has gained recent attention, because IDEXX Laboratories now includes this analyte (proprietary enzyme-linked immunosorbent assay [ELISA]) on their equine serum biochemical profile report. SDMA is a stable and continually released end product of protein metabolism within all cells. Similar to inulin, SDMA is freely filtered across glomeruli and neither reabsorbed nor secreted by the tubules.[23] More than 90% of SDMA is excreted in urine, with the remainder degraded by an as yet uncharacterized enzymatic pathway.[30] A meta-analysis of 18 human studies showed high correlation between SDMA and other GFR estimates.[31] Similar to CysC, but unlike Cr, SDMA appears to be minimally affected by muscle mass, breed, age, or sex in humans or small animals.[23,32] SDMA appears to be most useful as an earlier indicator of CKD in small animals, because serum concentration may increase with loss of only 40% of functional renal mass.[32] Furthermore, SDMA increased an average of 10 and 17 months earlier than Cr in dogs and cats, respectively, with spontaneous CKD.[33,34] Although SDMA concentrations increase in dogs with AKI, there are limited data to support SDMA as a superior measure to Cr in veterinary patients with AKI.[35]

Recently, Schott and colleagues[36] measured serum SDMA concentrations in 165 healthy competition draft horses of different breeds, ages, and sex. They found a strong correlation ($R = 0.72$, $P<.001$) between liquid chromatography-mass spectroscopy and IDEXX ELISA SDMA concentrations. The IDEXX ELISA was further validated by spike and recovery and dilutional parallelism studies. An upper reference limit of 14 μg/dL, as used for dogs and cats, was established for horses, with no apparent age (all animals were >6 months) or sex effects on SDMA concentrations.[36] Future evaluation of SDMA, compared with Cr, in horses with AKI and CKD is warranted.

Direct Measurement of Glomerular Filtration Rate

Several clearance techniques have been used experimentally to directly measure GFR in horses.[37–39] Unfortunately, these tests are cumbersome because they require bolus administration of a compound (classic is inulin) and serial blood sampling (to determine plasma clearance) or continuous rate infusion coupled with timed urine collections. However, determination of endogenous Cr clearance remains a simple and economic method to directly measure GFR. Using a collection device suspended below the prepuce (see **Fig. 2**) or bladder catheterization in mares, the volume of urine produced over 60 to 180 minutes can be readily determined. Measurement of Cr in a representative aliquot of total urine and a serum sample taken during the urine collection period allows calculation of endogenous Cr clearance:

$$\text{Clearance Cr (GFR, mL / kg / min)} = \left(\frac{[\text{Cr}]\text{urine}}{[\text{Cr}]\text{serum}} \times \text{urine output} \right) \Big/ \text{body weight (kg)}$$

Values for GFR in normal horses range from 1.5 to 3.0 mL/kg/min.[38]

Serum Electrolyte Concentrations

With decreased RBF, GFR, and UO consequent to hypovolemia, electrolyte concentrations should remain normal or increase, whereas hyponatremia and hypochloremia are characteristic findings in horses with AKI leading to acute renal failure.[40,41] Hyponatremia and hypochloremia are not specific for AKI, because they can be found in horses with GI disorders, for example, colitis. Serum potassium concentrations are variable in AKI, but substantial hyperkalemia (>6 mEq/L) is more common with oliguric to anuric AKI or uroperitoneum. Calcium and phosphate concentrations vary in horses with renal disease. Hypercalcemia and hypophosphatemia are often found in CKD, especially horses fed alfalfa hay, whereas hypocalcemia and hyperphosphatemia may be found with AKI. The combined findings of azotemia and hypercalcemia are essentially pathognomonic for CKD in horses.[22,42]

Other Serum Chemistry Values

Total protein concentration is often normal in horses with primary renal disease. In horses with AKI secondary to other disorders, total protein concentration is altered more by the primary disease than AKI. Some horses with chronic urinary tract inflammation (eg, pyelonephritis, cystitis) may have high globulin concentrations. With end-stage CKD, intestinal ulceration may result in hypoproteinemia. Mild hypoalbuminemia may develop with protein-losing glomerulopathies, and horses with primary glomerular disease may develop chronic hypoalbuminemia before onset of azotemia.[43]

Hematology

A minimum database for sick adult horses with suspected renal disease should include a complete blood count. High leukocyte counts and fibrinogen concentrations support an inflammatory process. Mild anemia (packed cell volume <28%) consequent to decreased erythropoietin production and a shortened erythrocyte lifespan with uremia may be observed in horses with CKD.[22] Administration of recombinant human or canine erythropoietin to horses with anemia of CKD is not recommended, because repeated dosing may lead to development of anti–erythropoietin antibodies.[44]

Acid-Base Balance

Venous blood gas analysis in horses with AKI usually reflects the primary disease, rather than the secondary renal insult. In the authors' experience, horses with colic are often mildly alkalotic from pain-induced hyperventilation. With more severe AKI and endotoxemia, a variable degree of lactic acidosis may be present. Horses with primary renal disease may have a mild metabolic acidosis, but acidosis is usually not severe until marked azotemia (Cr >10 mg/dL) develops with oliguric AKI or end-stage CKD.[14]

URINALYSIS
Gross Appearance

Color, clarity, odor, and turbidity should be evaluated at the time of collection. Normal equine urine is pale yellow to deep tan and often turbid from calcium carbonate crystals and mucus.[19] Toward the end of micturition or collection, urine may become milky white because of gravitation of crystals in the bladder.

Urine Tonicity

Although determination of USG with a refractometer is quick and easy (reagent strips should not be used to measure USG),[20] urine tonicity is more accurately determined by measurement of urine osmolality (U_{osm}). Larger molecules, such as glucose or proteins, can overestimate urine tonicity when assessed by specific gravity. Clinically, this is only a problem in patients with diabetes mellitus or heavy proteinuria, both of which are rare in horses. Use of refractometers with a wide specific gravity scale (1–1.06) is recommended to obviate extrapolating results for more concentrated urine, and the canine scale should be used with refractometers having separate canine and feline scales. The USG or U_{osm} is used to separate urine tonicity into 3 categories: (1) Urine more dilute than serum (hyposthenuria, USG <1.008 and U_{osm} <260 mOsm/kg); (2) Urine and serum of similar osmolality (isosthenuria, USG of 1.008–1.014 and U_{osm} of 260–300 mOsm/kg); and (3) Urine more concentrated than serum (USG >1.014 and U_{osm} >300 mOsm/kg).[20] Urine of normal horses consuming dry forage is usually concentrated (2–4 × serum tonicity) with a 1.025 to 1.040 USG and 600 to 1200 mOsm/kg U_{osm}, whereas pastured horses may have more dilute urine from high grass water content. Urine tonicity at hospital admission is an important criterion to determine AKI severity in dehydrated animals. With mild AKI, urinary concentrating ability may be retained with USG greater than 1.020 and U_{osm} greater than 500 mOsm/kg (values can be higher). With more severe AKI, urine concentrating ability is impaired with USG and U_{osm} typically less than 1.020 and 500 mOsm/kg, respectively, in the face of dehydration.[45]

Reagent Strip Analysis

Equine urine is usually alkaline (pH 8–9).[46] Strenuous exercise, metabolic acidosis, or bacteriuria can result in acidic pH, and urease-producing bacteria can impart a strong ammonia odor. Occasionally, aciduria is detected in anorectic horses with normal blood pH (eg, postoperative ileus with nasogastric reflux or enterocolitis). In these cases, "paradoxic" aciduria likely develops from potassium depletion and increased distal tubular hydrogen excretion (in exchange for potassium reabsorption).[47]

Urine reagent strips can yield false positive results for protein (trace to +) with alkaline samples, especially in concentrated urine.[48] However, a 2 to 3+ reaction for protein is usually supportive of proteinuria. Proteinuria can be specifically quantified on a chemistry analyzer and is usually less than 100 mg/dL in normal horses, resulting in a urine protein-to-creatinine ratio (UP:UCr) of less than 0.5,[49] whereas significant proteinuria from glomerulonephritis usually results in a UP:UCr greater than 2. Because proteinuria can accompany bacteriuria, pyuria, and hematuria, or may be found transiently following exercise,[50] an abnormal UP:UCr result must be interpreted considering these factors.

Normal equine urine should not contain glucose. Although the renal threshold for glucose has not been thoroughly evaluated in horses, early work indicated that it may be lower (160–180 mg/dL) than that of small animals and humans.[51] Glucosuria must always be interpreted with knowledge of serum/plasma glucose concentration. Hyperglycemia-associated glucosuria occurs with physiologic (eg, stress, exercise) and pathologic (eg, sepsis, pituitary pars intermedia dysfunction, diabetes mellitus) conditions or after administration of dextrose-containing fluids, parenteral nutrition, α_2-agonists, or corticosteroids.[17] When glucosuria is detected without hyperglycemia, proximal tubule dysfunction should be suspected. Glucosuria occurs more often in horses with AKI than CKD. Ketones are rarely detected in equine urine, even with advanced catabolic states or diabetes mellitus.

A positive result for blood on a urine reagent strip does not distinguish between hemoglobin, myoglobin, or intact red blood cells (RBC). Evaluation for hemolytic anemia with intravascular hemolysis (eg, hemoglobinemia), with muscle injury (eg, increased creatine kinase and aspartate aminotransferase activities), and of urine sediment for RBCs (or gross visualization of a centrifuged urine sample) can help differentiate between these pigments. Bilirubin reactions on reagent strips are often false positive reactions (eg, concentrated urine) but can occur with cholestatic liver disease.

Sediment Examination

Sediment examination remains an underutilized tool for evaluating urinary tract disorders in horses. Ideally, sediment should be examined within 30 to 60 minutes after collection. To perform sediment examination, 10 mL of fresh urine is centrifuged (usually in a conical plastic tube) at 300g for 3 to 5 minutes. The supernatant is discarded, and the pellet resuspended in the few drops of remaining urine. A drop of sediment is transferred to a glass slide and cover-slipped. The slide is examined at low magnification to evaluate for casts and crystals and at high magnification to quantify RBC, white blood cells (WBC), and epithelial cells, and to determine if bacteria are present.[19,20] Granular casts are rare in normal equine urine but can be seen with acute tubular injury. The numbers of granular casts per high-power field (hpf) can help differentiate transient from persistent AKI in people.[52] Casts are relatively unstable in alkaline urine; thus, sediment should be evaluated as soon as possible after collection. Normal urine contains less than 5 RBC or WBC/hpf and absent to rare bacteria. However, the lack of bacteria on sediment examination does not rule out urinary tract infection, and quantitative bacterial culture should be pursued when infection is suspected (eg, >5 WBC/hpf). Equine urine is rich in crystals, mostly variably sized calcium carbonate crystals, but calcium phosphate and calcium oxalate crystals can also be seen.[53,54] A few drops of 10% acetic acid solution may be added, if needed, to dissolve crystals if they obscure other sediment constituents.

URINE BIOCHEMICAL TESTS
Urine Electrolyte Clearance

Measurement of urine electrolyte clearances can yield useful information about tubular function/dysfunction with AKI and CKD. Because mammals evolved on a sodium-poor, potassium-rich diet, nephrons are more efficient in reabsorbing filtered sodium as compared with potassium. Horses with normal renal function can reabsorb greater than 99% of filtered sodium but only 85% to 90%, at most, of filtered potassium. Consequently, urine sodium concentration is usually low (<20 mmol/L) in horses fed an all forage diet, unless on salt supplementation, and urine potassium concentration is typically high (100–300 mmol/L).[38] With tubular injury and dysfunction, sodium reabsorption decreases and urine sodium concentration increases.[55] However, an increase in urine sodium concentration is not specific for tubular dysfunction because concentrations also increase with excess dietary salt intake or administration of sodium-rich intravenous or enteral fluids.[18,38] Thus, it can be challenging to determine whether increases in urine sodium concentration in sick horses are a consequence of AKI and tubular dysfunction or an appropriate response to sodium administration, unless urine assessment is performed before starting treatment.

Fractional electrolyte clearances can be measured to further assess tubular function, specifically, electrolyte resorption.[56,57] Fractional clearance is defined as the percentage of the filtered electrolyte that is excreted in urine and is calculated by dividing electrolyte clearance by Cr clearance (GFR):

$$\text{Electrolyte clearance (mL/min)} = \frac{[\text{electrolyte}]\text{urine}}{[\text{electrolyte}]\text{serum}} \times \text{urine output}$$

$$\text{Cr clearance (mL/min)} = \frac{[\text{Cr}]\text{urine}}{[\text{Cr}]\text{serum}} \times \text{urine output}$$

which, by rearrangement (canceling out UO) with expression as a percentage, becomes:

$$\text{Fractional electrolyte clearance}(\%) = \frac{[\text{electrolyte}]\text{urine}}{[\text{electrolyte}]\text{serum}} \times \frac{[\text{Cr}]\text{serum}}{[\text{Cr}]\text{urine}} \times 100\%$$

Fractional electrolyte clearances can be determined on a spot urine sample (voided or catheterized), without needing to measure UO with timed urine collection. Reference values for fractional electrolyte clearances in adult horses are provided in **Table 2**. Increased urine sodium concentration and fractional sodium clearance support tubular dysfunction, if measured before administration of sodium-rich solutions. In theory, the magnitude of increase in fractional sodium clearance should be proportional to the degree of tubular injury, although other factors (eg, tubular secretion of Cr, U_{osm}) may also affect calculated values. With AKI, horses with mild injury may continue to reabsorb greater than 99% of filtered

Table 2
Fractional electrolyte clearance (excretion) values for healthy adult horses

Electrolyte	Fractional Clearance, %	References
Sodium	<1	Morris et al,[56] 1984; Kohn & Strasser,[57] 1986
Chloride	<1.7	Morris et al,[56] 1984; Kohn & Strasser,[57] 1986
Potassium	24–75	Morris et al,[56] 1984; Kohn & Strasser,[57] 1986

sodium, and fractional sodium clearance will remain less than 1%, whereas values exceeding 10% may be found in horses with severe AKI.[45] Although increases in fractional sodium clearance can reflect tubular dysfunction, fractional potassium clearance is of value in assessing potassium balance. When horses are inappetent, fractional potassium clearance decreases, because of increased potassium reabsorption. However, mammalian kidneys do not have the same capacity to retain potassium, as compared with sodium, and ongoing UO results in further obligate losses (and body depletion) of potassium. In the authors' experience, fractional potassium clearance rarely drops to less than 15%, even in inappetent horses. Furthermore, during states of maximal potassium conservation, potassium can be resorbed in exchange with hydrogen in the distal tubule, leading to paradoxic aciduria as a simple proxy measurement supporting total body potassium depletion. With CKD, tubular compensation results in fractional electrolyte clearances remaining near normal values.

Enzymuria

Increased activities of proximal tubular epithelial brush border enzymes, specifically gamma glutamyl transferase (GGT), in urine supports tubular injury in horses (and other species).[38] Urine GGT activity is expressed as a ratio to urine Cr (urine GGT/urine Cr) with values >25 U/g considered increased.[38] It is a sensitive test, with urine GGT activity increasing 2 to 4 days before serum Cr in horses with gentamicin-induced proximal tubular injury.[58] Urinary GGT activity measurement is no longer commonly performed, because many clinicians deem the test "too sensitive," because values often increase reversibly in horses being treated with gentamicin for various infections.[59,60]

Biomarkers of Tubular Injury

There is considerable interest in identifying novel serum and urine markers to detect renal injury, before serum Cr increases or other measures of decreased renal function develop. In humans and small animals, the list of investigated biomarkers is long, but few are commercially available as diagnostic tests.[23,61–63] Novel biomarkers investigated in horses include neutrophil gelatinase-associated lipocalin (NGAL) and matrix metalloproteases-2 (MMP-2) and -9 (MMP9).[29,64] NGAL is a 178-amino-acid protein originally isolated from neutrophils but found in other tissues, including renal tubules. Within hours after kidney injury, NGAL production is upregulated in renal tubules, and serum and urine concentrations rapidly increase.[65] NGAL appears to be an extremely sensitive marker of renal injury, with serum concentrations increasing in proportion to severity of kidney damage and decreasing in parallel with improvement in renal function after treatment.[66] Using a commercial porcine-specific NGAL ELISA validated for equine serum, 1 study found concentrations of 7.4 to 103.6 µg/L and 9.8 to 2537 µg/L in normal horses and horses with high serum Cr, respectively.[64] In 1 small study, serum Cr concentration and urinary MMP-9, but not MMP-2, activity was higher in horses with colic undergoing abdominal surgical exploration versus horses undergoing castration. The investigators postulated that urinary MMP-9 may reflect renal injury.[29]

Although further work on novel biomarkers of renal function and injury in horses is needed, simple urine reagent strip analysis and measurement of urine enzyme activities remain viable tools for assessing AKI in horses. For example, detection of glucosuria on reagent strip analysis, in the face of normoglycemia, supports proximal tubule injury.

FUROSEMIDE STRESS TEST

In horses with oliguric AKI, intravenous administration of furosemide every 6 hours has been recommended to increase UO. However, anecdotally, this treatment is rarely effective.[38,67] A continuous rate of infusion of furosemide has been pursued for sustained renal delivery[68]; however, this treatment has not been critically evaluated in horses with AKI. In people, a furosemide stress test was developed to assess the short-term (2 hour) effect on UO. After baseline UO is determined (voiding or bladder catheterization), furosemide (1.0–1.5 mg/kg) is administered intravenously and UO is determined hourly for 2 to 6 hours.[69,70] In a small cohort of human patients with stage 1 AKI, this test was found to be a strong predictor of the reversibility of AKI (the greater the increase in UO, the more likely AKI was reversible). In fact, the test was a better predictor of AKI progression than several other traditional and novel urine biomarkers.[68] Evaluation of the furosemide stress test is warranted in horses.

REFERENCES

1. Macedo E, Mehta RL. Prerenal failure: from old concepts to new paradigms. Curr Opin Crit Care 2009;15:467–73.
2. Bellomo R, Ronco C, Kellum JA, et al. Acute renal failure–definition, outcome measures, animal models, fluid therapy and information technology needs: the Second International Consensus Conference of the Acute Dialysis Quality Initiative (ADQI) Group. Crit Care 2004;8:R204–12.
3. Mehta RL, Kellum JA, Shah SV, et al. Acute Kidney Injury Network: report of an initiative to improve outcomes in acute kidney injury. Crit Care 2007;11(1–8):R31.
4. McCullough PA, Kellum JA, Mehta RL, et al, Kidney Disease: Improving Global Outcomes (KDIGO) Acute Kidney Injury Work Group. KDIGO clinical practice guideline for acute kidney injury. Kidney Int Suppl 2012;2(1):1–138.
5. Chawla LS, Bellomo R, Bihorac A, et al. Acute kidney disease and renal recovery: consensus report of the Acute Disease Quality Initiative (ADQI) 16 Workgroup. Nat Rev Nephrol 2017;13:241–57.
6. Chertow GM, Burdick E, Honour M, et al. Acute kidney injury, mortality, length of stay, and costs in hospitalized patients. J Am Soc Nephrol 2005;16:3365–70.
7. Druml W, Lenz K, Laggner AN. Our paper 20 years later: from acute renal failure to acute kidney injury–the metamorphosis of a syndrome. Intensive Care Med 2015;41:1941–9.
8. Hoste EAJ, Kellum JA, Selby NM, et al. Global epidemiology and outcomes of acute kidney injury. Nat Rev Nephrol 2018;14:607–65.
9. Schott HC, Woodie JB. Diagnostic techniques and principles of urinary tract surgery. Chapter 64. In: Auer JA, Stick JA, Kümmerle JM, et al, editors. Equine surgery. 5th edition. St Louis (MO): Elsevier; 2019. p. 1095–114.
10. Chaney KP, Holcombe SJ, Schott HC, et al. Spurious hypercreatininemia: 28 neonatal foals (2000-2008). J Vet Emerg Crit Care 2010;20:244–9.
11. Groover ES, Woolums AR, Cole DJ, et al. Risk factors associated with renal insufficiency in horses with primary gastrointestinal disease: 26 cases (2000–2003). J Am Vet Med Assoc 2006;229:572–7.
12. Thoen ME, Kerl ME. Characterization of acute kidney injury in hospitalized dogs and evaluation of a veterinary acute kidney injury staging system. J Vet Emerg Crit Care 2011;21:648–57.
13. Savage VL, Marr CM, Bailey M, et al. Prevalence of acute kidney injury in a population of hospitalized horses. J Vet Intern Med 2019;330:2294–301.

14. Schott HC, Patterson KS, Fitzerald SD, et al. Chronic renal failure in 99 horses. In: Proceedings of the 43rd Annu Conv Am Assoc Equine Pract. Phoenix (AZ), December 1997. p. 345–6.

15. Website: IRIS Staging of CKD (modified 2019). International Renal Interest Society. Available at: http://www.iris-kidney.com/guidelines/staging.html. Accessed May 15, 2019.

16. Rumbaugh GE, Carlson GP, Harrold D. Urinary production in the healthy horse and in horses deprived of feed and water. Am J Vet Res 1982;43:735–7.

17. Thurmon JC, Steffey EP, Zinkl JG, et al. Xylazine causes transient dose-related hyperglycemia and increased urine volume in mares. Am J Vet Res 1984;45: 224–7.

18. Roussel AJ, Cohen ND, Ruoff WW, et al. Urinary indices of horses after intravenous administration of crystalloid solutions. J Vet Intern Med 1993;7:241–6.

19. Kohn CW, Chew DJ. Laboratory diagnosis and characterization of renal disease in horses. Vet Clin North Am Equine Pract 1987;3:585–615.

20. Wilson ME. Examination of the urinary tract in the horse. Vet Clin North Am Equine Pract 2007;23:563–75.

21. Braun JP, Lefebvre HP, Watson ADJ. Creatinine in the dog: a review. Vet Clin Pathol 2003;32:162–79.

22. Schott HC. Chronic renal failure in horses. Vet Clin North Am Equine Pract 2007; 23:593–612.

23. Hokamp JA, Nabity MB. Renal biomarkers in domestic species. Vet Clin Pathol 2016;45:28–56.

24. Ghys L, Paepe D, Smets P, et al. Cystatin C: a new renal marker and its potential use in small animal medicine. J Vet Intern Med 2014;28:1152–64.

25. Shlipak MG, Matsushita K, Ärnlöv J, et al. Cystatin C versus creatinine in determining risk based on kidney function. N Engl J Med 2013;369:932–43.

26. Zhang Z, Lu B, Sheng X, et al. Cystatin C in prediction of acute kidney injury: a systemic review and meta-analysis. Am J Kidney Dis 2011;58:356–65.

27. Safdar OY, Shalaby M, Khathlan N, et al. Serum cystatin is a useful marker for the diagnosis of acute kidney injury in critically ill children: prospective cohort study. BMC Nephrol 2016;17:130.

28. Qiu X, Liu C, Ye Y, et al. The diagnostic value of serum creatinine and cystatin C in evaluating glomerular filtration rate in patients with chronic kidney disease: a systematic literature review and meta-analysis. Oncotarget 2017;8:72985–99.

29. Arosalo BM, Raekallio M, Rajamäki M, et al. Detecting early kidney damage in horses with colic by measuring matrix metalloproteinase-9 and -2, other enzymes, urinary glucose and total proteins. Acta Vet Scand 2007;49:4.

30. Schwedhelm E, Böger RH. The role of asymmetric and symmetric dimethylarginines in renal disease. Nat Rev Nephrol 2011;7:275–85.

31. Kielstein JT, Salpeter SR, Bode-Böger SM, et al. Symmetric dimethylarginine (SDMA) as endogenous marker of renal function–a meta-analysis. Nephrol Dial Transplant 2006;21:2445–51.

32. Relford R, Robertson J, Clements C. Symmetric dimethylarginine: improving the diagnosis and staging of chronic kidney disease in small animals. Vet Clin Small Anim 2016;46:941–60.

33. Hall JA, Yerramilli M, Obare E, et al. Comparison of serum concentrations of symmetric dimethylarginine and creatinine as kidney function biomarkers in cats with chronic kidney disease. J Vet Intern Med 2014;28:1676–83.

34. Hall JA, Yerramilli M, Obare E, et al. Serum concentrations of symmetric dimethylarginine and creatinine in dogs with naturally occurring chronic kidney disease. J Vet Intern Med 2016;30:794–802.
35. Dahlem DP, Neiger R, Schweighauser A, et al. Plasma symmetric dimethylarginine concentration in dogs with acute kidney injury and chronic kidney disease. J Vet Intern Med 2017;31:799–804.
36. Schott HC, Gallant L, Coyne M, et al. Symmetric dimethylarginine and creatinine concentrations in draft horse breeds. J Vet Intern Med 2018;32:2128–9 [abstract].
37. Matthews HK, Andrews FM, Daniel GB, et al. Measuring renal function in horses. Vet Med 1993;88:349–56.
38. Schott HC, Waldridge B, Bayly WM. Disorders of the urinary system. Chapter 14. In: Reed SM, Bayly WM, Sellon DC, editors. Equine internal medicine. 4th edition. St Louis (MO): Elsevier; 2018. p. 888–990.
39. Lippi I, Bonelli F, Meucci V, et al. Estimation of glomerular filtration rate by plasma clearance of iohexol in healthy horses of various ages. J Vet Intern Med 2019;33: 2765–9.
40. Brobst DF, Grant BD, Hilbert BJ, et al. Blood biochemical changes in horses with prerenal and renal disease. J Equine Med Surg 1977;1:171–7.
41. Divers TJ, Whitlock RH, Byars TD, et al. Acute renal failure in six horses resulting from haemodynamic causes. Equine Vet J 1987;19:178–84.
42. LeRoy B, Woolums A, Wass J, et al. The relationship between serum calcium concentration and outcome in horses with renal failure presented to referral hospitals. J Vet Intern Med 2011;25:1426–30.
43. McSloy A, Poulsen K, Fisher PJ, et al. Diagnosis and treatment of a selective immunoglobulin M glomerulonephropathy in a quarter horse gelding. J Vet Intern Med 2007;21:874–7.
44. Piercy RJ, Swardson CJ, Hinchcliff KW. Erythroid hypoplasia and anemia following administration of recombinant human erythropoietin to two horses. J Am Vet Med Assoc 1998;212:244–7.
45. Grossman BS, Brobst DF, Kramer JW, et al. Urinary indices for differentiation of prerenal azotemia and renal azotemia in horses. J Am Vet Med Assoc 1982; 180:284–8.
46. Wood T, Weckman TJ, Henry PA, et al. Equine urine pH: normal population distributions and methods of acidification. Equine Vet J 1990;22:118–21.
47. Schott HC, Rossetto JR. Paradoxical aciduria in horses: 37 cases (2000-2008). J Vet Intern Med 2009;23:782.
48. Edwards DJ, Brownlow MA, Hutchins DR. Indices of renal function: reference values in normal horses. Aust Vet J 1989;66:60–3.
49. Uberti B, Eberle DB, Pressler BM, et al. Determination of and correlation between urine protein excretion and urine protein-to-creatinine ratio values during a 24-hour period in healthy horses and ponies. Am J Vet Res 2009;70:1551–6.
50. Schott HC, Hodgson DR, Bayly WM, et al. Haematuria, pigmenturia and proteinuria in exercising horses. Equine Vet J 1995;27:67–72.
51. Link RP. Glucose tolerance in horses. J Am Vet Med Assoc 1940;97:261–3.
52. Lima C, Macedo E. Urinary biochemistry in the diagnosis of acute kidney injury. Dis Markers 2018;2018:4907024.
53. Mair TS, Osborn RS. The crystalline composition of normal equine urine deposits. Equine Vet J 1990;22:364–5.
54. Neumann RD, Ruby AL, Ling GV, et al. Ultrastructure and mineral composition of urinary calculi from horses. Am J Vet Res 1994;55:1357–67.

55. Seanor JW, Byars TD, Boutcher JK. Renal disease associated with colic in horses. Mod Vet Pract 1984;65:A26–9.

56. Morris DD, Divers TJ, Whitlock RH. Renal clearance and fractional excretion of electrolytes over a 24-hour period in horses. Am J Vet Res 1984;45:2431–5.

57. Kohn CW, Strasser SL. 24-hour renal clearance and excretion of endogenous substances in the mare. Am J Vet Res 1986;47:1332–7.

58. Hinchcliff KW, McGuirk SM, MacWilliams PS, et al. Phenolsulfonphthalein pharmacokinetics and renal morphologic changes in adult pony mares with gentamicin-induced nephrotoxicosis. Am J Vet Res 1989;50:1848–53.

59. van der Harst MR, Bull S, Laffont CM, et al. Gentamicin nephrotoxicity–a comparison of in vitro findings with in vivo experiments in equines. Vet Res Comm 2005; 29:247–61.

60. Rossier Y, Divers TJ, Sweeney RW. Variations in urinary gamma glutamyl transferase/urinary creatinine ratio in horses with or without pleuropneumonia treated with gentamicin. Equine Vet J 1995;27:217–20.

61. Pressler BM. Clinical approach to advanced renal function testing in dogs and cats. Clin Lab Med 2015;35:487–502.

62. Rizvi MS, Kashani KB. Biomarkers for early detection of acute kidney injury. J Appl Lab Med 2017;2:386–99.

63. Kashani K, Cheungpasitporn W, Ronco C. Biomarkers of acute kidney injury: the pathway from discovery to clinical adoption. Clin Chem Lab Med 2017;26: 1074–89.

64. Jacobsen S, Berg LC, Tvermose E, et al. Validation of an ELISA for detection of neutrophil gelatinase-associated lipocalin (NGAL) in equine serum. Vet Clin Pathol 2018;47:603–7.

65. Mori K, Nakao K. Neutrophil gelatinase-associated lipocalin as the real-time indicator of active kidney damage. Kidney Int 2007;71:967–70.

66. Mishra J, Ma Q, Prada A, et al. Identification of neutrophil gelatinase-associated lipocalin as a novel early urinary biomarker for ischemic renal injury. J Am Soc Nephrol 2003;14:2534–43.

67. Geor RJ. Acute renal failure in horses. Vet Clin North Am Equine Pract 2007;23: 577–91.

68. Johansson AM, Gardner SY, Levince JF, et al. Furosemide continuous rate infusion in the horse: evaluation of enhanced efficacy and reduced side effects. J Vet Intern Med 2003;17:887–95.

69. Chawla LS, Davison DL, Brasha-Mitchell E, et al. Development and standardization of a furosemide stress test to predict the severity of acute kidney injury. Crit Care 2013;17:R207.

70. Koyner JK, Davison DL, Brasha-Mitchell E, et al. Furosemide stress test and biomarkers for the prediction of AKI severity. J Am Soc Nephrol 2015;26:2023–31.

Clinical Pathology of the Racehorse

Samuel D.A. Hurcombe, BSc, BVMS, MS

KEYWORDS

- Hematology • Hematocrit • Biochemistry • Troponin I • Lactate • Training
- Exercise • Performance

KEY POINTS

- Packed cell volume and hematocrit vary widely in response to training, disease and sympathoadrenal responses. The equine spleen holds up to 60% of erythrocyte mass.
- Cardiac troponin I is a useful biomarker of myocardial health. Assay-specific reference intervals should be considered when interpreting the results.
- Increases in gamma-glutamyl transferase activity have been associated with overtraining and seem to be unrelated to identified hepatotropic viruses in racehorses.
- Muscle enzymes activities can increase in response to training and subclinical and clinical myopathies. The magnitude of enzyme increase is proportional to the severity of injury.
- The time of sample acquisition in relation to exercise can affect clinical pathology results and should be taken into consideration when interpreting laboratory findings.

INTRODUCTION

This review focuses primarily on the Thoroughbred/Standardbred racehorse undergoing flat work. Horses in other disciplines, such as steeplechase and endurance racing, may share some similarities. Racing athletes must optimize their ability to supply oxygen (O_2) and other nutrients to tissues while simultaneously removing metabolic waste products. There have been several well-written book chapters and articles detailing clinical pathology of the equine athlete,[1,2] and the aim of this article is to provide recent information complementing previous work. A focus is placed on the assessment of clinicopathologic data in race horses and how factors such as training can affect adaptive responses that may both optimize performance and lead to laboratory derangements.

ERYTHRON AND OXYGENATION

Central to adequate tissue oxygenation and performance are erythrocytes containing hemoglobin. Simplistically, erythrocytes transport and deliver O_2 from the lungs to the

New Bolton Center, School of Veterinary Medicine, University of Pennsylvania, 382 West Street Road, Kennett Square, PA, USA
E-mail address: hurcombe@vet.upenn.edu

Vet Clin Equine 36 (2020) 135–145
https://doi.org/10.1016/j.cveq.2019.12.004
0749-0739/20/© 2019 Elsevier Inc. All rights reserved.

tissues for utilization. Erythrocytes are generated in the bone marrow by progenitor cells in response to erythropoietin (EPO). The average life span of a mature erythrocyte in circulation is 150 days, with approximately 250×10^6 circulating red cells dying per kilogram per hour.[3] Erythrocytes must be able to reversibly load O_2 in the pulmonary alveolus, unload O_2 at the tissue capillary interface, load carbon dioxide in the tissues, and unload carbon dioxide in the lungs. Central to this function is hemoglobin, a tetramer polypeptide (2 α chains and 2 β chains) with a central heme group that exhibits cooperative binding, wherein the affinity of hemoglobin for O_2 increases steadily as O_2 saturation goes from 0% to 100% for a given O_2 dissociation curve.

The O_2 dissociation curve (sometimes referred to as O_2 saturation curve) (**Fig. 1**), shows that when deoxygenated blood equilibrates gas mixtures of increasing the partial pressure of O_2 (P_{O2}), the binding sites for O_2 will become progressively occupied until, at a high enough P_{O2}, all of them will contain O_2. The curve is sigmoid in shape and is highly nonlinear in the normal physiologic range of P_{O2} (ie, 40–100 mm Hg). The middle portion of the curve (20%–80% saturation) is steeper than the low and high P_{O2} segments. Factors that influence O_2 binding to hemoglobin and the position of the O_2 dissociation curve include 2,3 diphosphoglycerate (2,3 DPG), pH, temperature, and

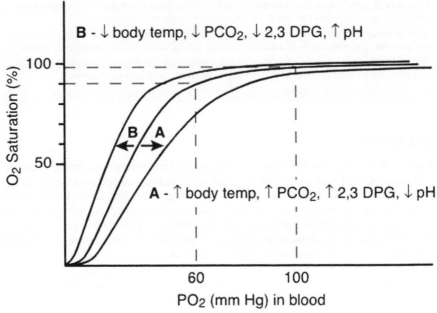

Fig. 1. O_2–hemoglobin dissociation curve. The O_2 saturation (the percentage of hemoglobin in the oxyhemoglobin state) is plotted as a function of P_{O2}. Note the sigmoid shape of the curve. Above a partial pressure of about 60 mm Hg, the curve is relatively flat, with O_2 saturations of greater than 90%. Below a P_{O2} of 60 mm Hg, the O_2 saturation decreases rapidly (ie, the O_2 comes off the hemoglobin). The P_{O2} of 100 mm Hg shown on the graph corresponds with a normal alveolar P_{O2} (at sea level) and translates to an O_2 saturation of nearly 100%. Factors that shift the curve to the right include increased body temperature, increased partial pressure of carbon dioxide, increased 2,3 DPG, and decreased pH. Factors that shift the curve to the left include decreased body temperature, decreased partial pressure of carbon dioxide, decreased 2,3 DPG, and increased pH. (*From* Schwartzstein RM, Parker MJ: *Respiratory physiology: a clinical approach,* Philadelphia, 2006, Lippincott Williams & Wilkins, p 109; with permission.)

partial pressure of carbon dioxide. These factors are allosteric effectors and a rightward shift owing to increases in temperature and partial pressure of carbon dioxide or decreases in 2,3 DPG or pH cause a decreased O_2 affinity for hemoglobin and promote unloading of O_2 to the tissues at the expense of adenosine triphosphate production (termed 2,3 DPG shunt or the Rapaport-Luebering cycle).[3] The opposite effect occurs with decreasing temperature and partial pressure of carbon dioxide or increases in 2,3 DPG and pH. This phenomenon is also termed the Bohr effect. These effects are particularly relevant in the exercising athlete, where a rightward shift allows for easier unloading of O_2 to tissues.[3]

FACTORS AFFECTING THE HEMOGRAM

In horses, a relationship exists between red blood cell volume, training, and performance, where red blood cell mass increases in response to training and age and is correlated with racing performance.[4] The changes in red blood cell indices associated with intense exercise occur to accommodate the delivery of greater than 80 L of O_2 per minute to the tissue of a fit Thoroughbred racehorse during maximal activity.[5]

Intense exercise has been associated with increased red blood cell fragility with subsequent liberation of hemoglobin leading to increased unconjugated bilirubin concentrations. As pH decreases owing to lactic acid production and temperature increases with thermogenesis, the red blood cell membrane becomes fragile.[6] Red cells may also become echinocytic with exercise and postulated to be due to adenosine triphosphate depletion and ionic shifts, but the exact cause is unclear. These cells can be recognized on a blood smear.[7]

The equine spleen represents a significant erythrocyte reservoir (50%–60%) that is able to be mobilized to increase the effective circulating red blood cell mass.[3,8] Excitement or apprehension can lead to increases in packed cell volume (PCV or hematocrit [HCT]) or a relative erythrocytosis of up to 0.25 L/L (25%) via catecholamine-mediated splenic contraction. Moreover, the excitement associated with simply walking to the racecourse can increase PCV by 0.60 to 0.13 L/L in racehorses.[9] The PCV increases may then take at least 2 hours to return to baseline values after exercise or excitement.[10] This characteristic can make the interpretation of PCV/HCT, hemoglobin concentration, and red blood cell counts challenging, because these tests may not fully represent the actual red blood cell volume. Another major confounding factor in assessing red blood cell concentrations in exercised horses is the change in plasma volume, with fluid shifting extravascularly, resulting in an increase in plasma protein concentration and PCV after racing (upwards of a 10% change in individual animals), thereby affecting maximal PCV assessments.[11]

Breed differences exist between Standardbred and Thoroughbred racehorses and their red blood cell content. Standardbreds have a total blood volume of 121 mL/kg versus 142 mL/kg in Thoroughbreds. However, total plasma volume is similar between the 2 breeds.[4] Generally, Thoroughbreds have higher PCV, maximal PCV (after exercise), and hemoglobin concentration compared with Standardbreds.[1]

Training effects on PCV and total red blood cell mass have also been observed in racehorses. Changes in red blood cell mass were most obvious in the early training period (first 7 weeks) compared with training periods beyond 7 weeks where no significant increases were observed.[12] Mechanisms for this increase in PCV are not well-understood. One proposed mechanism is exercise-induced arterial hypoxemia with subsequent stimulation of erythropoiesis, yet this is unsubstantiated.[5]

Diet may affect the hemogram and can be of notable relevance in racehorses. Feeding of hay is associated with fluid shifts to the gut compared with grain feeding, resulting in increases in HCT and total protein that remain high for several hours.[13] This effect is amplified further if a large meal is provided compared with multiple smaller feedings throughout the day.[14]

ANEMIA IN RACEHORSES

Anemia, characterized by a low PCV/HCT, hemoglobin concentration, and/or total red blood cell count, may be caused by several factors. Typically, the average racehorse, in training or racing, has a higher resting PCV than a more sedentary horse. As such, anemia may be relative where the actual measured PCV may be within a normal established reference interval yet is inappropriately low for an athlete. Decreased or decreasing PCV (nonregenerative anemia of inflammatory/chronic disease) has been associated with viral respiratory disease,[15,16] a common occurrence among intensively housed young Thoroughbred and Standardbred horses at track barns.

Erythropoietin Administration

There are sporadic reports of human recombinant EPO (rhEPO) administration in horses causing nonregenerative anemia through the development of anti-EPO antibody production.[17,18]

McKeever[19] showed that exogenous EPO administration resulted in an 18% increase in hemoglobin concentration and PCV, a 20% increase in Vo_{2max}, and a 17% increase in the content of arterial blood O_2 in splenectomized Standardbred racehorses. There is no doubt that stimulation of bone marrow by EPO is performance enhancing. The study further showed that EPO resulted in increased performance as measured by total running time compared with control horses.

Piercy and colleagues[17] demonstrated marked erythroid hypoplasia with high myeloid to erythroid ratios in the bone marrow of 2 horses administered rhEPO repeatedly. Serum from affected horses inhibited rhEPO-induced proliferation of erythroid progenitors in vitro. It was presumed that the developed anti-rhEPO antibodies cross-reacted with endogenous EPO, thereby inhibiting erythropoiesis.[18] Multiple blood transfusions were palliative in a Thoroughbred racehorse with rhEPO-induced nonregenerative anemia, but ultimately the horse died.[19] As such, rhEPO should not be administered to horses to boost erythrocyte values or treat anemia.

Iron Status in Horses

True iron deficiency as a cause of anemia in the performance horse is rare. Despite this, it remains a common concern of trainers and veterinarians. Ferritin, as a marker of iron status, was measured in Standardbreds, Finnhorses, and half-bred riding horses after moderate exercise on a racetrack, treadmill, and/or race. Exercise increased plasma ferritin proportionally to the intensity of exercise and returned to baseline at rest, which may be an acute phase response. Owing to these changes, Hyyppa and colleagues[20] suggested basal ferritin concentration should be measured after at least 2 days of rest after strenuous exercise. Importantly, because ferritin is a positive acute phase protein, changes in the serum ferritin concentration should be interpreted in conjunction with other markers of inflammation.

LEUKON RESPONSES IN THE RACEHORSE

Leukogram alterations in response to training have been reported in horses. Strenuous exercise can cause a mild physiologic lymphocytosis, which is usually transient.[21,22] Cortisol-induced stress leukogram responses are also transient and characterized by a mature neutrophilia (no band cells/left shift) and lymphopenia.[23] This finding may be explained by sympathoadrenal responses on the spleen ejecting a reservoir pool of neutrophils as well as the effects of corticosteroids and catecholamines on recruiting marginated neutrophils in circulation.[10,15] Moreover, approximately 50% of the total mature neutrophil numbers reside within the splenic pulp/sinusoids and capillary blood.[24] Overtraining has been associated with eosinopenia and an increased neutrophil:lymphocyte ratio has been observed in response to long-term training.[12] Wong and colleagues[25] showed that, after a single strenuous exercise test, serum cortisol concentrations increased as well as the neutrophil:lymphocyte ratio. Furthermore, neutrophil function may also be transiently impaired as evidenced by altered chemotactic locomotion and reduced oxidative burst activity in horses after exercise.

PLASMA PROTEIN RESPONSES TO EXERCISE

Exercise induces rapid shifts and redistribution of fluid and electrolytes within body compartments resulting in a decrease in plasma volume after exercise. These changes are proportional to the duration and intensity of exercise. The resultant plasma volume contraction results in relative erythrocytosis and an increase in plasma protein concentration (globulins and albumin) for upwards of 1 hour. Ambient conditions may also contribute to further insensible losses of fluid through breath water and sweat.[2,17]

CARDIAC BIOMARKERS IN RACEHORSES

Cardiac troponin I (CTnI) is a cardiac muscle–specific biomarker that can increase in response to myocardial inflammation, ischemia, and workload.[26] The magnitude of injury is correlated with the magnitude of CTnI increase. Moreover, specific to exercising horses, CTnI may increase with endurance racing and short-term strenuous treadmill exercise. Nostell and Haggstrom[27] evaluated CTnI concentrations in healthy Standardbred, Thoroughbred, and Warmblood horses at rest and in a smaller subset of Standardbred and Thoroughbred racehorses after racing under field conditions (with no standardization of pace or distance). In that study, the majority of horses did not have significant increases in CTnI after race work, a finding corroborated elsewhere.[28] However, 1/17 Standardbred and 2/6 Thoroughbred horses had mild but significant increases at 1 to 2 hours after the race and 4/21 Standardbred and 1/6 Thoroughbred horses had similar increases at 10 to 14 hours after a race, indicating that exercise can increase CTnI activity in some horses.[27]

Rossi and colleagues[29] evaluated the magnitude and time course of CTnI release and clearance after maximal effort in normal Standardbred racehorses undertaking a controlled near-race intensity exercise trial using 2 different CTnI assays. Their exercise protocol consisted of more than 15 minutes of a warmup jog on a dirt training track (mean, 28.8 minutes) followed by 1 mile at submaximal intensity (mean, 2:09 minutes) and then cool down of light jogging/walking. The resting mean CTnI was 1.38 ± 0.6 ng/L. All horses showed an increase after exercise with peak concentrations occurring 2 to 6 hours after exercise (11.96 ± 9.41 ng/L). Based on sequential sampling, the half-life for endogenous CTnI was calculated to be 6.4 hours. Interestingly, this finding is in contrast with a study in ponies, where recombinant equine CTnI was administered and found to have a half-life of 0.47 hours.[30] Differences in the proportion of horses with elevations in CTnI after exercise between studies exist likely owing to numbers of subjects, type of exercise conditions tested, and breed of horse.[27,29] The clinical significance of the increase in CTnI in response to exercise is not known and its association with other commonly diagnosed cardiac conditions in racehorses has not been fully elucidated. For example, horses with lone atrial fibrillation, a common performance limiting dysrhythmia in Thoroughbred and Standardbred racehorses associated with increased atrial myocardial workload, rarely have increases in CTnI concentrations.[31] The exact mechanisms for CTnI increases in response to exercise in some horses are poorly understood, but are likely relate to the location of myocardial injury (atrial vs ventricular), duration of injury (prolonged vs transient), and type of injury (inflammatory vs ischemic) among others. CTnI obtained at rest or postexercise challenge may be a useful adjunctive test in cases of poor performance where primary or secondary cardiac disease are suspected. Certainly, if a significant murmur or dysrhythmia is found, CTnI concentrations may be beneficial and can be used to assess response to therapy.

Another cardiac biomarker, measurement of the myocardial isoenzyme of creatine kinase myocardial band activity has been suggested in horses; however, the greatest creatine kinase myocardial band activity occurs in splenic and intestinal tissue; therefore, it is not specific for cardiac disease.[32,33]

MARKERS OF HEPATOBILIARY FUNCTION AND DYSFUNCTION IN RACEHORSES

Gamma glutamyl transferase (GGT) activity has been evaluated in racehorses where increases have been associated with both cumulative days in training[12] as well as poor performance.[34] Mild increases in GGT and total bilirubin concentration (unconjugated fraction) have been observed in seemingly healthy horses in training and are presumed to be a physiologic response to training by unknown mechanisms.[35] More recently, 4 hepatotropic viruses have identified in horses. These have been investigated as a possible cause for hepatobiliary enzyme activity increases and even clinical disease in horses. Specifically, hepacivirus A, pegivirus E, pegivirus D (also termed Theiler's disease-associated virus), and equine parvovirus may be detected in blood using RNA or DNA (virus-dependent) molecular techniques.

Ramsay and colleagues[36] recently reported the prevalence of increased GGT and-sorbitol dehydrogenase (SDH) activities in racing Thoroughbreds and the association between increased enzyme activities and the detection of hepatotropic viruses. More than 800 racing Thoroughbreds in California had prerace bloods evaluated for GGT and SDH activities and nucleic acid presence for all 4 viruses. Of these horses, 19% had increased GGT activity with 2% being greater than twice the upper reference limit (40 IU/L). Furthermore, almost one-half of the horses (46.9%) had increased SDH activity with 6% being greater than twice the upper reference limit (7 IU/L). The prevalence of virus detection in their population was 18.2% for pegivirus A, 2.5% for hepacivirus A, 0.5% pegivirus D, and 2.9% for parvovirus. However, a statistical association between high GGT and/or SDH activities with hepatotropic virus detection was not found.[36]

At this time, the significance of increased serum GGT activity beyond being a marker of training intensity in athletic horses remains unclear. Increases in hepatocellular leakage enzymes should be evaluated in context of the horses' clinical findings. The presence of icterus, behavioral changes, inappetence, and weight loss may indicate significant liver disease and warrants further investigation. Further studies are needed to determine the significance, if any, of hepatotropic viruses and a potential link with increases in GGT activity in racehorses.

MUSCLE ENZYME ACTIVITIES IN RACEHORSES

Myopathies are a common cause of poor performance in racehorses. Exertional rhabdomyolysis and polysaccharide storage myopathy are 2 conditions affecting primarily the skeletal muscle of the horse.[37] Creatine kinase, specifically the skeletal muscle isoenzyme creatine kinase MM and aspartate aminotransferase (AST) activities increase rapidly in response to muscle trauma, inflammation, and necrosis. Each enzyme has uniquely specific kinetics in the body. Creatine kinase activity peaks by 4 to 6 hours from the onset of damage and has a half-life of approximately 2 hours.[38] If the insult is transient in nature, creatine kinase activity falls rapidly.[39] The activity of AST, however, peaks approximately 12 to 24 hours after muscle or liver injury in the horse. Activities are slower to return to normal after even a transient insult owing to the longer half-life of 7 to 8 days.[39] It is important to remember that AST is found in the cytosol and mitochondria of hepatocytes and is therefore a nonspecific indicator of skeletal muscle damage. Thus, the interpretation of creatine kinase and AST activities should be done with consideration to other biochemical indicators of liver status, particularly other liver leakage enzymes, such as SDH, and glutamate dehydrogenase, but also GGT activity and total bilirubin concentration. For example, increased AST and creatine kinase activities and no alterations in SDH, glutamate dehydrogenase, or GGT activities supports the AST being of muscle origin. Moreover, modest and very high increases in creatine kinase activity are often observed in horses with myopathic disorders, both at rest and after exercise. For example, creatine kinase activity in horses with polysaccharide storage myopathy or exertional rhabdomyolysis can easily reach more than 10,000 U/L and more than 1,000,000 U/L, respectively. Lactate dehydrogenase is also not specific for muscle injury and is found in muscle, the liver, and red blood cells.

Brief periods of maximal exercise lead to mild increases in creatine kinase and AST activity, whereas submaximal exercise should not result in enzyme activity increases. In normal horses at maximum exercise, these increases should rarely exceed a few hundred units per liter.[40] Unlike other species, exercising horses can increase AST activity upwards of 30%. In early training, resting activities are 50% to 100% greater than that of horses not in training.[41] The magnitude of increase in muscle enzymes in racehorses can be extremely variable and a function of several factors, including genetics, presence of heritable myopathy, level of fitness, recent diet, and degree of workload, to name a few. With a mild but persistent increase in creatine kinase/AST activities in response to submaximal exercise or simply at even rest, these findings should raise the index of suspicion the potential of an underlying muscle disorder. A controlled exercise challenge test consisting of 12 to 15 minutes of trotting exercise and evaluating creatine kinase and AST activities before and after exercise can be valuable in identifying a muscle disorder in equine athletes. A 2- to 4-fold increase in creatine kinase activity after 4 hours rest is suggestive of a myopathy, even if no other overt clinical signs are present (ie, muscle stiffness, tachycardia, sweating, pain).[42] Overtraining also causes increases in resting AST activity compared with control horses. Clinically, overtraining can result muscle damage as shown in 1 study where some exercised horses on an incline treadmill developed gluteal muscle atrophy.[1]

LACTATE AND RACEHORSES

L-Lactate is produced from anaerobic glycolysis and is an expected response in the context of exercise because both aerobic and anerobic pathways to produce adenosine triphosphate are used.[43] Point-of-care testing availability makes lactate assessment accessible in both the field and the hospital setting, using handheld readers. Whole blood is recommended for lactate assessment[1] in the horse because plasma lactate concentrations can be up to 1.5 times higher than that of whole blood. Discrepancies exist owing to variable uptake of lactate by erythrocytes.[44]

The rate of lactate production and accumulation can be influenced by many factors, but the speed at which the horse works significantly determines lactate production.

Speeds of more than 7 to 9 m/s herald the onset of rapid lactate production and accumulation, also termed onset of blood lactate accumulation (OBLA) or when blood lactate reaches 4 mmol/L (V4).[45] The speed at which lactate reaches 4 mmol/L is also termed the lactate threshold or aerobic–anaerobic threshold and is a useful indicator of aerobic capacity.[46] Lactate concentrations can exceed 25 mmol/L during intense exercise and, on a short-term basis, horses have a remarkable ability to buffer and metabolize acute sharp increases in lactate. The OBLA has been proposed to be an indicator of fitness or marker of effectiveness of the training program. Speed at OBLA depends on several factors. Inherent fitness, level of training, gait, breed of horse, and diet all influence OBLA. Typically, if blood lactate concentration is plotted against speed, fitter horses accumulate lactate at higher speeds (rightward curve shift) than less fit horses. Several studies have confirmed that a higher V4 is associated with superior performance.[46,47] The OBLA is potentially more useful as a marker of fitness for horses competing at greater distances or longer races vs sprinters. Typically, stayers may rely more on their aerobic capacity to yield energy for the demands of a sustained exercise vocation.[1,48]

TIMING OF SAMPLING

A 2018 study assessed albumin, cholesterol, creatinine, creatine kinase, AST, lactate dehydrogenase, GGT, calcium, phosphate, magnesium, sodium, potassium, cortisol, HCT, hemoglobin, red blood cell count, white blood cell count, neutrophil count, and lymphocyte count in Standardbred racehorses serially before and after racing.[49] They assessed variables at 3 and 2 days before a race as well as 2 and 3 days after race. Horses ran at a mean speed of 12.9 m/s for an average of 1959 m. Plasma calcium concentrations were lower at 3 days after the race compared with 2 days before the race and phosphate concentrations and GGT activities were higher 2 and 3 days after the race compared with prerace timepoints. The HCT, red blood cell counts, and hemoglobin concentrations were higher 2 days after the race compared with prerace timepoints and 3 days after the race. No other significant differences were found. The authors suggest that these data highlight the importance of timing and sampling. Most variables had returned to baseline (prerace) levels by 2 days after the race.[49] Other studies suggest that, in Thoroughbreds, levels may take 3 days or longer to return to baseline, notably enzyme activities for creatine kinase, lactate dehydrogenase, GGT, and AST (up to 5 days).[50]

SUMMARY

The assessment of a complete blood count and serum biochemical panel in racehorses can provide useful data on performance and health status. Adaptive responses to training and workload must be considered when interpreting results. Reference intervals from most laboratories do not reflect a racing or training horse population exclusively, so the practitioner should be aware of expected changes in response to exercise in these animals when interpreting clinicopathologic findings. Biomarkers of health, performance and recovery in human athletes such as insulin-like growth factor 1, sex hormone concentrations and their precursors, total iron binding capacity, inflammatory cytokines (IL-6 and IL-8), and S-100 calcium binding protein B have yet to be investigated in equine athletes.[51]

DISCLOSURE

The author has nothing to disclose.

REFERENCES

1. McGowan C. Clinical pathology in the racing horse: the role of clinical pathology in assessing fitness and performance in the racehorse. Vet Clin Equine 2008;24: 405–21.
2. McKenzie EC. Hematology and serum biochemistry of the equine athlete, chapter 42. In: Hinchcliff K, editor. Equine sports medicine and surgery. 2nd edition. St Louis (MO): Saunders Ltd; 2014. p. 921–9.
3. Stockham SL, Scott MA. Erythrocytes, chapter 3. In: Scott MA, editor. Fundamentals of veterinary clinical pathology. 2nd edition. Ames (IA): Blackwell Publishing; 2008. p. 110–211.
4. Persson SGB. Blood volume, state of training and working capacity of racehorses. Equine Vet J 1968;1:52–62.
5. Poole DC, Erickson HE. Cardiovascular function and oxygen transport: responses to exercise and training. In: Hinchcliff KW, Geor RJ, Kaneps AJ, editors. Equine exercise physiology – the science of exercise in the athletic horse. Philadelphia: Elsevier Limited; 2008. p. 212–45.
6. Hanzawa K, Kai M, Hirage A, et al. Fragility of red cells during exercise is affected by blood pH and temperature. Equine Vet J Suppl 1999;30:610–1.
7. Poso AR, Soveri T, Oksanen HE. The effect of exercise on blood parameters in standardbred and Finnish-bred horses. Acta Vet Scand 1983;24(2):170–84.
8. Persson SG, Ekman L, Lyndin G, et al. Circulatory effects of splenectomy in the horse. II. Effect of plasma volume and total and circulating red cell volume. Zentralbl Veterinarmed A 1973;20:456–68.
9. Revington M. Haematology of the racing Thoroughbred in Australia 1: reference values and the effect of excitement. Equine Vet J 1983;15:141–4.
10. Snow DH. Physiological factors affecting resting haematology. In: Snow DH, Persson SGB, Rose RJ, editors. Equine exercise physiology. Cambridge (MA): Granata editions; 1983. p. 318–23.
11. Persson SGB. The significance of haematological data in the evaluation of soundness and fitness in the horse. In: Snow DH, Persson SGB, Rose RJ, editors. Equine exercise physiology. Cambridge (MA): Granata editions; 1983. p. 324–7.
12. Tyler-McGowan CM, Golland LC, Evans DL, et al. Haematological and biochemical responses to training and overtraining. Equine Vet J Suppl 1999;30:621–5.
13. Kerr MG, Snow DH. Alterations in plasma proteins and electrolytes in horses following the feeding of hay. Vet Rec 1982;110:538–40.
14. Clarke LL, Ganjam VK, FichtenbaumB, et al. Effect of feeding on renin-angiotensin-aldosterone system of the horse. Am J Physiol 1988;254:R524–30.
15. Carlson GP. Haematology and body fluids in the equine athlete: a review. In: Gillespie JR, Robinson NE, editors. Equine exercise physiology 2. Davis (CA): ICEPP Publications; 1987. p. 393–425.
16. Kannegieter NJ, Frogley A, Crispe E, et al. Clinical outcomes and virology of equine influenza in a naïve population and in horses infected soon after receiving one dose of vaccine. Aust Vet J 2011;89(suppl 1):139–42.
17. Piercy RJ, Swardson CJ, Hinchcliff KW. Erythroid hypoplasia and anemia following administration of recombinant human erythropoietin to two horses. J Am Vet Med Assoc 1998;212:244–7.
18. Woods PR, Campbell G, Cowell RL. Nonregenerative anaemia associated with administration of recombinant human erythropoietin to a Thoroughbred racehorse. Equine Vet J 1997;29:326–8.

19. McKeever KH. Body fluids and electrolytes. In: Hinchcliff KW, Geor RJ, Kaneps AJ, editors. Equine exercise physiology – the science of exercise in the athletic horse. Philadelphia: Elsevier Limited; 2008. p. 328–49.

20. Hyyppa S, Hoyhtya M, Nevalainen M, et al. Effect of exercise on plasma ferritin concentrations: implications for the measurement of iron status. Equine Vet J 2002;34:186–90.

21. Rose RJ, Allen JR, Hodgson DR, et al. Responses to submaximal treadmill exercise and training in the horse: changes in haematology, arterial blood gas and acid base measurements, plasma biochemical values and heart rate. Vet Rec 1983;113(26–27):612–8.

22. Snow DH, Ricketts SW, Mason DK. Haematological response to racing and training exercise in Thoroughbred horses, with particular reference to the leucocyte response. Equine Vet J 1983;15(2):149–54.

23. Donovan DC, Jackson CA, Colahan PT, et al. Assessment of exercise-induced alterations in neutrophil function in horses. Am J Vet Res 2007;68:1198–204.

24. Carakostas MC, Moore WE, Smith JE. Intravascular neutrophilic granulocyte kinetics in horses. Am J Vet Res 1981;42:623–5.

25. Wong CW, Smith SE, Thong YH, et al. Effects of exercise stress on various immune functions in horses. Am J Vet Res 1992;53:1414–7.

26. Babuin L, Jaffe AS. Troponin: the biomarker of choice for the detection of cardiac injury. CMAJ 2005;173:1191–202.

27. Nostell K, Haggstrom J. Resting concentrations of cardiac troponin I in fit horses and effect of racing. J Vet Cardiol 2008;10:105–9.

28. Begg LM, Hoffman KL, Begg AP. Serum and plasma cardiac troponin I concentrations in clinically normal Thoroughbreds in training in Australia. Aust Vet J 2006;84:336–7.

29. Rossi TM, Kavsak PA, Maxie MG, et al. Post-exercise cardiac troponin I release and clearance in normal Standardbred racehorses. Equine Vet J 2019;51:97–101.

30. Kraus MS, Kaufer BB, Damiani A, et al. Elimination half-life of intravenously administered equine cardiac troponin I in healthy ponies. Equine Vet J 2013; 45:56–9.

31. Jesty SA, Kraus MS, Gelzer AR, et al. Effect of transvenous cardioversion on plasma cardiac troponin I concentrations in horses with atrial fibrillation. J Vet Intern Med 2009;23:1103–7.

32. Argiroudis SA, Kent JE, Blackmore DJ. Observations on the isoenzymes of creatine kinase in equine serum and tissue. Equine Vet J 1982;14:317–21.

33. Tsung SH. Several conditions causing elevation of serum CK-MB and CK-BB. Am J Clin Pathol 1981;75:711–5.

34. Snow DH, Gash SP, Rice D. Field observations on selenium status, whole blood glutathione peroxidase and plasma gamma glutamyl transferase activities in Thoroughbred racehorses. In: Gillespie JR, Robinson NE, editors. Davis(CA): Equine Exercise Physiology 2; ICEEP 1987. p. 494–505.

35. Allen BV, Powel DG. Effects of training and time of day on blood sampling on the variation of some common haematological parameters in normal Thoroughbred racehorses. In: Snow DH, Persson SGB, Rose RJ, editors. Equine exercise physiology. Cambridge (United Kingdom): Granta Editions; 1983. p. 328–53.

36. Ramsay JD, Evanoff R, Mealey RH, et al. The prevalence of elevated gamma-glutamyltransferase and sorbitol dehydrogenase activity in racing Thoroughbreds and their associations with viral infection. Equine Vet J 2019;51(6):738–42.

37. Martin BB Jr, Reef VB, Parente EJ, et al. Causes of poor performance of horses during training, racing, or showing: 348 cases (1992-1996). J Am Vet Med Assoc 2000;216:554–8.
38. Volfinger L, Lassourd V, Michaux JM, et al. Kinetic evaluation of muscle damage during exercise by calculation of amount of creatine kinase released. Am J Physiol 1994;266:434–41.
39. Stockham SL, Scott MA. Enzymes, chapter 12. In: Scott MA, editor. Fundamentals of veterinary clinical pathology. 2nd edition. Ames (IA): Blackwell Publishing; 2008. p. 640–69.
40. Harris PA, Marlin DJ, Gray J. Plasma aspartate aminotransferase and creatine kinase activities in Thoroughbred racehorses in relation to age, sex, exercise and training. Vet J 1998;155:295–304.
41. eClinPath, Cornell University College of Veterinary Medicine. Available at: www.eclinpath.com. Accessed March 15, 2019.
42. MacLeay JM. Disorders of the musculoskeletal system. In: Reed SM, Bayly WM, Sellon DC, editors. Equine internal medicine. 3rd edition. St Louis (MO): Saunders Elsevier; 2010. p. 488–544.
43. Saibene F, Cortili G, Gavazzi P, et al. Maximal anaerobic (lactic) capacity and power of the horse. Equine Vet J 1985;17:130–2.
44. Koho NM, Vaihkonen LK, Poso AR. Lactate transport in red blood cells by monocarboxylate transporters. Equine Vet J Suppl 2002;34:555–9.
45. Thornton J, Essen-Gustavsson B, Linholm A, et al. Effects of training and detraining on oxygen uptake, cardiac output, blood gas tensions, pH and lactate during and after exercise in the horse. In: Snow DH, Persson SGB, Rose RJ, editors. Equine exercise physiology. Cambridge (MA): Granata editions; 1983. p. 470–86.
46. Lindner AE. Relationships between racing times of Standardbreds and V4 and V200. J Anim Sci 2010;88:95–954.
47. Courouce A, Chatard JC, Auvinet B. Estimation of performance potential of Standardbred trotters from blood lactate concentrations measured in field conditions. Equine Vet J 1997;29:365–9.
48. Harris RC, Marlin DJ, Snow DH. Metabolic response to maximal exercise of 800 and 2000 m in the Thoroughbred horses. J App Physiol 1987;63:12–9.
49. Bos A, Compagnie E, Lindner A. Effect of racing on blood variables in Standardbred horses. Vet Clin Pathol 2018;47:625–8.
50. Sommer H, Szemes Am, Felbinger U. Effect of racing on enzymes and metabolites in blood serum of Thoroughbred racehorses. Tierarztl Umsch 1982;37:751–9.
51. Lee EC, Fragala MS, Kavouras SA, et al. Biomarkers in sports and exercise: tracking health, performance, and recovery in athletes. J Strength Cond Res 2017;31:2920–37.

Equine Inflammatory Markers in the Twenty-First Century: A Focus on Serum Amyloid A

Alicia Long, DVM, Rose Nolen-Walston, DVM*

KEYWORDS

- Serum amyloid A • Acute phase protein • Fibrinogen • Inflammation • Equine
- Horse

KEY POINTS

- Serum amyloid A (SAA) is the only major acute phase protein in the horse, with concentrations increasing rapidly after an inflammatory stimulus up to high levels compared with baseline, with a subsequent rapid decrease following cessation of the inflammatory process.
- Serum amyloid A is a more sensitive marker of inflammation than other more commonly evaluated laboratory parameters (eg, fibrinogen and white blood cell count).
- Multiple different inflammatory and infectious conditions result in an increase in serum amyloid A levels, including but not limited to colitis, pneumonia, reproductive disease, and septic arthritis.
- Elevations in SAA are not specific for a certain disease process and can increase with inflammation in the absence of infection; elevations in SAA should be evaluated in conjunction with physical examination findings and results of other diagnostic tests.

A continuing challenge faced by veterinary practitioners is early identification of illness, with the goal to initiate early treatment to improve outcome. Patients in early stages of disease can have subtle enough abnormalities that differentiating them from healthy animals is difficult; therefore, sensitive methods to identify diseased patients are desirable. This is particularly true in diseases involving inflammation and infection, where early intervention can affect short- and long-term prognosis. In addition, diagnostic modalities that allow for monitoring of treatment response are extremely useful for guiding therapeutics and assessing prognosis.

Acute phase proteins (APP) are blood proteins synthesized mainly by hepatocytes and are a part of the acute phase response (APR) of the innate immune system.[1–3]

Department of Clinical Studies, New Bolton Center, 382 West Street Road, Kennett Square, PA 19348, USA
* Corresponding author.
E-mail address: rnolenw@upenn.edu

Vet Clin Equine 36 (2020) 147–160
https://doi.org/10.1016/j.cveq.2019.12.005
0749-0739/20/© 2020 Elsevier Inc. All rights reserved.

APP are classified as either negative or positive, depending on whether their serum/plasma levels decrease or increase during an APR, respectively. A notable negative APP is albumin, with positive APP including fibrinogen, haptoglobin, and serum amyloid A (SAA). Serum/plasma levels of positive APP increase in response to a triggering event (eg, infection, trauma) and decrease coinciding with recovery; the magnitude of increase and rate of decline varies between species and the specific APP.[3]

Equine SAA is an apolipoprotein consisting of three isoforms and is complexed primarily to high-density lipoproteins.[4-6] Mainly produced by the liver, extrahepatic secretion of SAA also occurs into colostrum and synovial fluid. SAA is the only major positive APP in the horse. A major APP is defined as one whose concentrations are low or clinically undetectable in normal animals but rapidly increase greater than 10-fold during the APR and rapidly decrease with disease resolution. Relapse or a new/secondary insult result in a return to increased concentrations.[4] This contrasts with moderate APPs, such as fibrinogen and haptoglobin in the horse, which are detectable in serum/plasma of healthy animals, have a slower response to stimuli, and increase 1- to 10-fold during the APR. Fibrinogen has remained the mainstay of blood analysis for inflammation in horses and other large animal species, largely because of the ease and minimal expense of testing. However, fibrinogen concentrations do not increase for 24 hours after the inciting inflammatory event and only peak at 48 to 72 hours.[7] Additionally, the increase in fibrinogen concentrations is small (usually 1- to 2-fold) making it difficult to reliably detect mild inflammation. In contrast, serum/plasma SAA concentrations increase up to 1000 times as soon as 6 hours after stimulation and, once the stimulus is removed, concentrations decrease within 12 hours because of its short half-life (30–120 minutes).[5,8,9]

The widespread use of fibrinogen versus SAA measurement in large animals most likely started as a function of assay availability. Methods of diagnostic evaluation of SAA have greatly improved since its discovery as a major APP, allowing for inexpensive testing in serum or plasma stallside or in laboratories.[10-13] SAA is stable at room temperature and refrigerated, allowing for transport before testing[10] and can be measured in noninvasive samples, such as saliva.[14] Although there are differences in precision and accuracy between assays, most available tests seem accurate enough within clinically relevant ranges.[8,10,11,13] Various publications refer to SAA in mg/L, μg/mL, and ng/mL; the first two of these units are equivalent and the third represents one thousandth the concentration of the first.

SERUM AMYLOID A IN NORMAL HORSES COMPARED WITH HORSES WITH INFECTIOUS OR INFLAMMATORY DISEASE

A commonly accepted reference interval for SAA concentration in horses is 0 to 20 mg/L,[15] with most reports finding normal horses have SAA values at or lower than 12 mg/L.[6,8,16-30] Several studies have examined the utility of SAA for discriminating between horses with or without inflammation. Animals with systemic inflammation had significantly higher SAA concentrations (mean, 1583 mg/L; range, 688–4000 mg/L) than horses with local or no inflammation (mean of 343 mg/L and range of 37–1609, and mean of 5.6 mg/L and range of 1.8–14.5 mg/L, respectively). This discrimination was more distinct than that of fibrinogen, where the mean concentrations of the three groups were 224, 181, and 128 mg/dL, respectively.[31] For differentiating clinically normal horses from those with infectious or inflammatory disease, SAA measurement had a sensitivity of 53%, specificity of 94%, and diagnostic accuracy of 75%, whereas white blood cell count, plasma fibrinogen concentrations, and albumin/globulin ratios had lower diagnostic accuracy (59%–62%).[32] In cases where serial SAA measurements were obtained, horses with increasing SAA concentrations between 24 and 72 hours of admission were significantly more likely to develop complications or be euthanized, whereas there was no significant difference in outcome in horses with increased SAA concentrations at admission.[25]

SERUM AMYLOID A IN FOALS

Multiple reports have shown foals have similar baseline values of SAA to adult horses and the rate of rise and fall is comparable between foals and adults.[33–36] Foals with sepsis and other bacterial infections have significantly higher SAA concentrations than healthy foals or sick foals without inflammation, although there is enough overlap in the concentrations among these groups that SAA should not be used as a sole means of identifying infection or sepsis.[35–38] In the largest study evaluating SAA in foals, a healthy control group of 226 Thoroughbred neonates had median SAA concentrations of 0.9, 4.5, and 2.5 mg/L on 1, 2, and 3 days old, with the values on Day 2 being significantly higher than on Day 1.[33] In 136 foals with clinical disease, median SAA concentrations of cases with focal infections (eg, omphalitis) were 195 mg/L and those with septicemia higher still at 280 mg/L. Foals with noninflammatory abnormalities, such as failure of passive transfer and noninfectious disease, had low SAA concentrations at 5.1 and 3.1 mg/L, respectively. A separate small study found that foals with positive blood cultures had markedly increased SAA concentrations compared with foals with ambiguous or negative blood cultures, which had moderate or no increases in SAA concentrations, respectively.[35]

Because of the presence of SAA within colostrum, it has been suggested that the increased SAA concentrations in normal foals shortly after birth may be associated with colostral absorption.[39] High fibrinogen levels in neonatal foals can often indicate intrauterine inflammation. Although less is known about SAA levels with intrauterine inflammation, one report assessing the relationship between intrauterine or umbilical cord bacteria with foal health following parturition found no significant difference between postpartum SAA levels and the presence of bacteria in amniotic fluid or venous umbilical blood.[40]

GASTROINTESTINAL DISEASE AND SERUM AMYLOID A

In regards to colic, multiple different APPs have been evaluated for their ability to distinguish surgical from medical causes of colic, and their usefulness in monitoring for complications and predicting prognosis and response to treatment. Most[4,41,42] but not all[43,44] studies have found that SAA concentrations are significantly higher (median, 65[41] to 935 mg/L[42]) in horses with colic-attributable inflammatory causes (eg, enteritis, colitis, peritonitis, or abdominal abscesses) versus surgical and noninflammatory colic (median, 4.8[41] to 228 mg/L[42]). Furthermore, SAA concentrations were increased in horses with equine grass sickness (median, 50 mg/L) compared with those with surgical and noninflammatory colic (median, ~0 mg/L).[45] In contrast to these reports, one prospective study found that 62% of horses with colic requiring surgical intervention had SAA concentrations greater than or equal to 5 mg/L, compared with 19% of medically managed horses, although cases of peritonitis or colitis were excluded.[43] A smaller retrospective study also found that SAA concentrations did not distinguish between surgical and nonsurgical or strangulating and nonstrangulating lesions.[44]

Several studies have shown that peritoneal fluid SAA concentrations are increased in horses with colic compared with control horses, although peritoneal fluid concentrations are not higher than that in serum/plasma.[42,46,47] However, peritoneal fluid SAA concentrations increase more rapidly in horses with strangulating lesions than other diseases, although it only discriminated between simple obstruction and strangulating or inflammatory colics of greater than 24 hours duration.[47]

It is known that surgery itself, such as exploratory celiotomy for colic, causes an increase in APPs, including SAA.[43,48–50] Compared with more minor surgical procedures, exploratory celiotomy causes a prolonged APR, with serum SAA concentrations increased from 48 to 96 hours after surgery (compared with 12–24 hours with minor procedures).[48,50,51] Horses with postoperative complications had a more pronounced increase in SAA (61.4-fold over baseline) and took longer to achieve peak values (96 hours) compared with horses without complications (29-fold increase; peak at 48 hours).[50] Another prospective study assessing SAA and complications in postoperative colic patients found that the magnitude of SAA increase was greater at 48 hours and 4 to 6 days postsurgery in horses with versus those without complications.[49]

The data are conflicting regarding the accuracy and utility of SAA for determining outcome and prognosis in horses with colic. One study[44] found no significant differences in SAA concentration between survivors and nonsurvivors, whereas another larger study[50] of horses undergoing exploratory celiotomy found that patients with increased SAA concentrations 5 days postoperatively were slightly less likely to survive to discharge (odds ratio, 0.97). Taken together, the current literature with equine colic suggests that SAA alone does not offer clear guidance on differentiating surgical from nonsurgical colics nor should it be relied on for prognosticating survivability when euthanasia is being considered. However, colic cases that are admitted with higher SAA concentrations ($\geq$20, and typically 60–1000 mg/L) should have inflammatory lesions, such as enteritis and colitis, higher on the differential diagnostic list.

There are fewer available studies assessing SAA in gastrointestinal diseases other than colic. A small experimental study found that inoculation with equine *Coronavirus* resulted in SAA concentrations that mirrored naturally occurring disease; although all three challenged horses shed large quantities of virus, only those that showed clinical signs of diarrhea, fever, and anorexia had increased SAA concentrations, which peaked at 200 to 400 g/L.[21]

SERUM AMYLOID A AND EQUINE RESPIRATORY DISEASES

SAA has been investigated mainly for its ability to distinguish infectious from noninfectious causes of respiratory disease and to separate horses with bacterial pneumonia from those with viral infections. Several studies have demonstrated that transport alone, the major risk factor for pneumonia in horses, can cause increased SAA concentrations, ranging from around 30 to 500 µg/mL for 24 to 48 hours after long-distance (1200 km) shipping.[52] This increase was significantly diminished by administration of antimicrobials[52,53] but shorter transport times (4 hours) had no effect.[54]

Horses naturally infected with equine influenza virus A2 (H3N8) had increased SAA concentrations during the first 48 hours of clinical signs. Concentrations then returned to baseline within 11 to 22 days.[55] A useful characteristic of SAA is that it does not increase higher than baseline in horses naturally exposed to but not infected with equine herpes virus type 1 or *Streptococcus equi* subsp *equi*.[29] In bacterial pneumonia, marked increases in SAA concentrations is seen (in the thousands)[32] and one prospective study found that the SAA concentration correlated better with rectal temperature and clinical resolution of disease than fibrinogen concentrations in Thoroughbreds experimentally infected with *S equi* subsp *zooepidemicus*.[16] Concentrations of SAA peaked at Day 3 postinoculation and returned to baseline at Day 15 as compared with fibrinogen, which peaked at Days 4 to 5 and returned to baseline by

Day 22. Concentrations of SAA in horses were significantly lower in horses with equine influenza virus and equine herpes virus type 1 infection (median, 731 mg/L and 1173 mg/L, respectively; range, 0 to ≥3000 mg/L) than those positive for S equi subsp equi (median, 1953 mg/L; range, 0 to ≥3000 mg/L). Because of the significant overlap between horses with viral and bacterial respiratory disease, SAA concentrations alone cannot be used to distinguish between these two groups.[30]

When examining horses with equine asthma (separated into inflammatory airway disease or recurrent airway obstruction in the highlighted studies), multiple investigations have found increases in SAA concentration in affected horses compared with control subjects.[19,26] In contrast, other studies found no significant differences in SAA concentrations in horses with inflammatory airway disease or recurrent airway obstruction and control horses.[56,57] Therefore, the main utility of SAA measurement in equine asthma seems to be differentiating these cases from horses with infectious respiratory disease.

RHODOCOCCUS EQUI AND SERUM AMYLOID A

Some of the challenges with Rhodococcus equi include identifying subclinically affected foals before they develop clinical disease and determining which patients will benefit from antibiotic treatment, especially with issues of antimicrobial resistance. Several studies have investigated SAA as a possible predictor of R equi pneumonia in at-risk populations. The first study used a large, well-selected population of affected foals and age-matched control animals from endemic farms.[58] No predictive value for the incidence of pneumonia was found in SAA concentrations in 212 foals between 7 and 14 days old or 196 foals between 21 and 28 days of age nor in the onset of clinical signs of pneumonia. The authors concluded that "monitoring concentrations of SAA is not useful as a screening test for early detection of R equi."[58] A subsequent smaller study that assessed weekly screening with SAA to identify preclinical R equi infections in an endemic farm diagnosed with R equi pneumonia found similar results.[59] In the latter study, SAA concentrations were not associated with the development of sonographic evidence of lung abscessation and only two of six foals with pneumonia had high SAA concentrations.

Another more recent study investigated APPs in foals with bronchopneumonia caused by various pathogens, including R equi. In foals on a farm with endemic R equi infection, no correlation was seen between SAA concentrations and the radiographic score of foals who developed R equi pneumonia. The ability of SAA to predict development of R equi in foals using a cutoff point of greater than 53 μg/mL was found to be limited (sensitivity, 64%; specificity, 77%).[37] The limited utility of SAA in identifying preclinical cases of R equi is surprising because this organism generally yields robust increases in fibrinogen concentrations and leukocyte count, which are less sensitive than SAA for detection of other inflammatory diseases. No definitive answer for this discrepancy has been elucidated.

SURGERY AND SERUM AMYLOID A

Even minor surgical procedures cause inflammation and this is reflected in multiple reports that have demonstrated increases in SAA concentrations following elective procedures.[29,34,51,55] Recognizing that SAA can increase postsurgery is important, but serial measurement of SAA may be a useful early marker of horses with postoperative infections. In a study of horses after castration,[60] all horses had high SAA concentrations (around 400–600 mg/L) at Day 3 postoperatively, but those that developed infections still had SAA values in this range on the eighth day, whereas horses recovering without complication had lower concentrations (around 200 mg/L). The infections were not reliably reflected by increases in rectal temperature, leukocyte count, or fibrinogen concentration, suggesting that SAA was a superior marker for infection. A subsequent study found that SAA concentrations increased in horses undergoing castration but those given perioperative penicillin and flunixin versus flunixin alone had lower SAA concentrations on Days 3 (515 mg/L vs 708 mg/L) and 8 (125 vs 545 mg/L) postcastration,[61] suggesting that mild subclinical infections after surgery result in appreciable differences in SAA concentration.

With other minor surgical procedures, peak SAA concentrations of 100 to 400 mg/L approximately 3 days after surgery is expected in cases uncomplicated by infection. Concentrations of SAA were also significantly lower in elective (defined as noninflamed) versus nonelective (preexisting inflammatory foci) cases.[34] Measurement of SAA was also able to delineate differing levels of surgical trauma based on invasiveness.[51] In several of these studies[34,51] the SAA response was found to be a more sensitive indicator of inflammation than various other APP or leukocyte responses, and concentrations dropped quicker than fibrinogen with resolution. This is particularly useful to the practitioner who must decide whether hematologic evidence of inflammation is simply a holdover from effects of surgery or indicative of postoperative infection that requires further diagnostic evaluation or treatment.

SERUM AMYLOID A IN REPRODUCTIVE HEALTH AND DISEASE

There are conflicting data on SAA concentrations in the periparturient period of healthy mares. One study found that SAA levels remained low in the 8-week prepartum period with slight increases in some mares in the last week before foaling.[20] Two other studies found no increases in SAA concentration before parturition.[62,63] Healthy mares do show increases in SAA concentration in the 24 to 36 hours following parturition, which return to baseline values 5 to 7 days postpartum[20,62]; in one study, the mean SAA concentration reached 62 mg/L (range, 0.7–305 mg/L) and 189 mg/L (range, 0–1615 mg/L) at 12 and 36 hours postpartum, respectively.[20]

Most reports have found no changes in serum SAA concentrations following breeding or infectious endometritis.[22,28,64,65] Only one study showed a significant increase in serum APP levels (SAA and fibrinogen) after experimental induction of endometritis.[66] Based on these results, measurement of SAA concentrations does not seem to be useful for endometritis assessment in horses.

Mares who experienced early embryonic death versus healthy control mares were more likely to have SAA concentrations greater than 30 mg/L.[18] Some mares in the early embryonic death group had increased SAA concentrations before ovulation (mean, 687 mg/L) that remained high until 10 days postovulation. The authors hypothesized that the mares with increased SAA concentrations before ovulation had undiagnosed endometritis before breeding.[18]

In mares with experimentally induced placentitis, SAA concentrations peaked between 274 and 4385 mg/L within 2 to 6 days after intracervical inoculation; mares generally aborted within 2 to 6 days of the initial rise in SAA greater than the reference interval.[20,63] Abortion was more likely in mares with high SAA concentrations compared with mares with SAA concentrations within the reference interval,[20] and values in the former group increased steadily until abortion, after which they rapidly decreased. In comparison, fibrinogen concentrations and white blood cell counts were not found to be useful markers of placentitis.[63] A prospective study examining fetal serum samples found that SAA concentrations were significantly increased in cases where a causative microorganism was identified and either fetal multiorgan disease (10–40 mg/L) or placentitis (2.5 to >40 mg/L) was present, compared with cases of placentitis without an identifiable microorganism or in which no infectious or inflammatory cause was found (<2.5 mg/L).[67]

SERUM AMYLOID A AND DISEASES OF EQUINE JOINTS AND SYNOVIAL STRUCTURES

A comparatively large amount of literature is available regarding SAA concentrations in septic arthritis and tenosynovitis and, overall, SAA seems to be a sensitive marker of these diseases in adult horses. Healthy control horses have serum and synovial concentrations of SAA that are generally less than 1 mg/L. Repeated arthrocentesis (which increases the nucleated cell count and total protein) and intra-articular amikacin injection do not affect SAA concentrations and SAA measurement in these cases may be important because the effects of repeated sampling can confound assessment of treatment efficacy and resolution.[68,69] Additionally, more recent studies have found that repeated arthroscopy and repeated through-and-through joint lavage also do not affect synovial or serum SAA concentrations, whereas the nucleated cell count and total protein are increased following these procedures alone.[70,71] Although most of the SAA found within synovial fluid may be an ultrafiltrate from plasma, a joint-specific isoform of SAA is produced by synoviocytes.[72]

As in other diseases, bacterial infection of joints and other synovial structures seems to be the most potent stimulant of SAA production. Concentrations of SAA in plasma and synovial fluid are increased in horses with septic synovial disease (synovial fluid, mean of 39.2 mg/L and range of 0–368.9 mg/L; plasma, mean of 275.5 mg/L and range of 0–1421.8 mg/L) but not nonseptic (synovial fluid, mean of 0 mg/L and range of 0–29.7 mg/L; plasma, mean of 0.5 mg/L and range of 0–17 mg/L) or control groups.[73] A study examining SAA in experimentally induced inflammatory synovitis and septic arthritis found similar differences between groups in serum and synovial fluid SAA concentrations.[74] For the septic and aseptic groups, the mean peak synovial SAA concentrations were 135 mg/L (range, 60–555 mg/L) and 0 µg/L (range, 0–0), respectively, whereas the mean peak serum SAA concentrations were 663 mg/L (range, 217–1434 mg/L) and 0 mg/L (0–0), respectively. This study did find a delayed increase in synovial (no appreciable increase until 36 hours, at which time it peaked) compared with serum (began to increase at 24 hours, peaked at 36 hours) SAA concentrations after induction of septic synovitis.[74]

Horses with penetrating wounds to a synovial structure that presented within 24 hours after the initial injury had lower plasma SAA concentrations at admission (median, 23 mg/L) and a faster decrease following surgery, compared with horses requiring multiple surgeries, which had a median SAA concentration of 3378 mg/L at admission, with persistent increases 48 hours postoperatively (median, 2525 mg/L).[75]

LAMINITIS, OBESITY, AND SERUM AMYLOID A

Determining how SAA concentrations change in laminitis is complicated by the myriad of inflammatory and noninflammatory causes, and the variable chronicity and severity of the disorder. Additionally, conflicting data exist regarding the role of obesity and inflammation within horses. Concentrations of SAA were not increased in previously laminitic ponies that were in remission, but exercise caused slight increases in some ponies.[76,77] In obese equids, increases in SAA concentrations were correlated with higher body condition score and higher plasma insulin concentrations.[78] However, the SAA concentrations in all of the horses were within the reference interval

(3.8 mg/L was the highest result), so the diagnostic utility of using SAA to assess for inflammation in obese horses is uncertain.[78]

EXERCISE AND SERUM AMYLOID A

Several observational studies have evaluated the effects of long-distance rides in horses.[17,79,80] In endurance horses, SAA concentrations significantly increased (10-fold) from baseline after long-distance, but not after limited-distance, races.[80] Arabian horses that were just beginning endurance training had higher SAA concentrations versus baseline compared with experienced horses undergoing the same effort.[79] However, SAA concentrations increased similarly postrace in experienced and inexperienced horses.[17] Prerace SAA concentrations were significantly lower in Arabian endurance horses that finished the race versus those who could not complete the distance.[17]

A study of racing Standardbred trotters found that acute strenuous exercise did not cause significant increases in SAA concentration[81] and there was only a weak correlation between SAA concentration and cumulative training days in training thoroughbreds followed for several months of training.[82] Overall, SAA concentrations seem to increase to a greater degree with endurance exercise as compared with short-distance (including strenuous) work, with variations between types of exercise likely being subtle enough to make clinical utility of these findings minimal.

SERUM AMYLOID A AND PARASITES

In a study of horses experimentally infected with small and large strongyles, APPs were monitored over 161 to 164 days. Although haptoglobin and iron concentrations and albumin/globulin ratios were associated with strongyle burden, SAA concentrations were not and remained low throughout the study.[83] Additionally, no significant changes in SAA concentration were seen after anthelmintic treatment in two separate groups of experimentally infested and heavily parasitized horses.[84,85] This provides the practitioner with useful information because larval cyathostomiasis is a difficult diagnosis to make antemortem, and low SAA concentrations are uncommon with inflammatory colonopathies.

SERUM AMYLOID A AND VACCINATION

After vaccination with two different influenza and tetanus toxoid products, horses showed variable APRs with SAA concentrations increasing higher than 5 mg/L and peaking (~30–175 mg/L) at 48 hours after vaccination in 6/10 horses. Increased white blood cell counts, fibrinogen concentrations, and decreased serum iron concentrations were also noted. By 96 hours, SAA concentrations declined but had not quite reached baseline values.[86]

OTHER DISEASES AND SERUM AMYLOID A LEVELS

One prospective study evaluated horses with ocular disease (ulcerative keratitis) as compared with two control groups (positive control horses with systemic inflammation but no ocular disease and negative control horses with no evidence of ocular or systemic disease).[87] Compared with the negative control group, positive control horses, but not the ocular disease group, had significantly higher fibrinogen and SAA. The authors concluded that increases in APPs in patients with ocular disease should raise suspicion for systemic inflammation.

A retrospective study assessed the usefulness of SAA in the diagnosis of equine protozoal myeloencephalitis using stored serum or cerebrospinal fluid samples from 25 clinical cases.[88] Affected horses had low or undetectable SAA concentrations in both sample types, indicating that SAA measurement is unlikely to aid in a clinical diagnosis of this disease.

SUMMARY

SAA is a sensitive predictor of early inflammation and, because of its rapid onset and short half-life, tracks the course of disease closely. In most studies, it outperforms the other commonly used markers of inflammation, fibrinogen and white blood cell count, and also seems superior to the other acute phase markers, including haptoglobin, C-reactive protein, and serum/plasma iron. However, it is not useful to diagnose specific diseases and should not replace careful physical examination or diagnostic testing to identify of the cause of the inflammatory response.

Although SAA has many advantages, it is still not a diagnostic panacea. It seems to have limited validity in screening foals for R equi pneumonia, although it often increases to extremely high concentrations in pleuropneumonia in adult horses and is valuable in assessing response to treatment in such cases. SAA also does not reliably distinguish surgical from nonsurgical colic cases and, although it may possibly be oversensitive, serial testing of SAA is likely superior to that of fibrinogen in identifying postoperative infections. Any deviations from a steady fall after the first 2 to 3 days after surgery might prompt a search for infectious complications. Overall, practitioners should feel comfortable using SAA in lieu of fibrinogen (and certainly in preference to complete blood count (CBC), in the authors' opinion) for most cases where infectious or inflammatory disease is suspected, although measuring both initially may be useful for the practitioner with limited experience in interpreting the wide range of results with this marker.

DISCLOSURE

The authors have nothing to disclose.

REFERENCES

1. Cray C, Zaias J, Altman NH. Acute phase response in animals: a review. Comp Med 2009;59(6):10.
2. Eckersall PD, Bell R. Acute phase proteins: biomarkers of infection and inflammation in veterinary medicine. Vet J 2010;185(1):23–7.
3. Petersen HH, Nielsen JP, Heegaard PMH. Application of acute phase protein measurements in veterinary clinical chemistry. Vet Res 2004;35(2):163–87.
4. Crisman MV, Scarratt WK, Zimmerman KL. Blood proteins and inflammation in the horse. Vet Clin North Am Equine Pract 2008;24(2):285–97, vi.
5. Tape C, Kisilevsky R. Apolipoprotein A-I and apolipoprotein SAA half-lives during acute inflammation and amyloidogenesis. Biochim Biophys Acta 1990;1043(3):295–300.
6. Hultén C, Sletten K, Foyn Bruun C, et al. The acute phase serum amyloid A protein (SAA) in the horse: isolation and characterization of three isoforms. Vet Immunol Immunopathol 1997;57(3):215–27.
7. Borges AiS, Divers TJ, Stokol T, et al. Serum iron and plasma fibrinogen concentrations as indicators of systemic inflammatory diseases in horses. J Vet Intern Med 2007;21(3):489–94.

8. Jacobsen S, Kjelgaard-Hansen M, Hagbard Petersen H, et al. Evaluation of a commercially available human serum amyloid A (SAA) turbidometric immuno-assay for determination of equine SAA concentrations. Vet J 2006;172(2):315–9.

9. Nunokawa Y, Fujinaga T, Taira T, et al. Evaluation of serum amyloid A protein as an acute-phase reactive protein in horses. J Vet Med Sci 1993;55(6):1011–6.

10. Hillström A, Tvedten H, Lilliehöök I. Evaluation of an in-clinic serum amyloid A (SAA) assay and assessment of the effects of storage on SAA samples. Acta Vet Scand 2010;52:8.

11. Christensen M, Jacobsen S, Ichiyanagi T, et al. Evaluation of an automated assay based on monoclonal anti-human serum amyloid A (SAA) antibodies for mea-surement of canine, feline, and equine SAA. Vet J 2012;194(3):332–7.

12. Howard J, Graubner C. Comparison of paired serum and lithium heparin plasma samples for the measurement of serum amyloid A in horses using an automated turbidimetric immunoassay. Vet J 2014;199(3):457–60.

13. Schwartz D, Pusterla N, Jacobsen S, et al. Analytical validation of a new point-of-care assay for serum amyloid A in horses. Equine Vet J 2018;50(5):678–83.

14. Jacobsen S, Top Adler DM, Bundgaard L, et al. The use of liquid chromatography tandem mass spectrometry to detect proteins in saliva from horses with and without systemic inflammation. Vet J 2014;202(3):483–8.

15. Witkowska-Piłaszewicz OD, Żmigrodzka M, Winnicka A, et al. Serum amyloid A in equine health and disease. Equine Vet J 2019;51(3):293–8.

16. Hobo S, Niwa H, Anzai T. Evaluation of serum amyloid a and surfactant protein d in sera for identification of the clinical condition of horses with bacterial pneu-monia. J Vet Med Sci 2007;69(8):827–30.

17. Cywinska A, Gorecka R, Szarska E, et al. Serum amyloid A level as a potential indicator of the status of endurance horses: serum amyloid A in endurance hors-es. Equine Vet J 2010;42:23–7.

18. Krakowski L, Krawczyk CH, Kostro K, et al. Serum levels of acute phase proteins: SAA, Hp and progesterone (P4) in mares with early embryonic death. Reprod Domest Anim 2011;46(4):624–9.

19. Lavoie-Lamoureux A, Leclere M, Lemos K, et al. Markers of systemic inflamma-tion in horses with heaves. J Vet Intern Med 2012;26(6):1419–26.

20. Coutinho da Silva MA, Canisso IF, MacPherson ML, et al. Serum amyloid A con-centration in healthy periparturient mares and mares with ascending placentitis. Equine Vet J 2013;45(5):619–24.

21. Nemoto M, Oue Y, Morita Y, et al. Experimental inoculation of equine coronavirus into Japanese draft horses. Arch Virol 2014;159(12):3329–34.

22. Tuppits U, Orro T, Einarsson S, et al. Influence of the uterine inflammatory response after insemination with frozen–thawed semen on serum concentrations of acute phase proteins in mares. Anim Reprod Sci 2014;146(3):182–6.

23. Back H, Penell J, Pringle J, et al. A longitudinal study of poor performance and subclinical respiratory viral activity in Standardbred trotters. Vet Rec Open 2015;2(1):e000107.

24. Cywińska A, Czopowicz M, Witkowski L, et al. Reference intervals for selected he-matological and biochemical variables in Hucul horses. Pol J Vet Sci 2015;18(2):439–45.

25. Westerman TL, Tornquist SJ, Foster CM, et al. Evaluation of serum amyloid A and haptoglobin concentrations as prognostic indicators for horses with inflammatory disease examined at a tertiary care hospital. Am J Vet Res 2015;76(10):882–8.

26. Bullone M, de Lagarde M, Vargas A, et al. Serum surfactant protein D and hapto-globin as potential biomarkers for inflammatory airway disease in horses. J Vet Intern Med 2015;29(6):1707–11.

27. El-Bahr SM, El-Deeb WM. Acute-phase proteins, oxidative stress biomarkers, proinflammatory cytokines, and cardiac troponin in Arabian mares affected with pyometra. Theriogenology 2016;86(4):1132–6.

28. Sikora M, Król J, Nowak M, et al. The usefulness of uterine lavage and acute phase protein levels as a diagnostic tool for subclinical endometritis in Icelandic mares. Acta Vet Scand 2015;58(1):50.

29. Pepys MB, Baltz ML, Tennent GA, et al. Serum amyloid A protein (SAA) in horses: objective measurement of the acute phase response. Equine Vet J 1989;21(2): 106–9.

30. Viner M, Mazan M, Bedenice D, et al. Comparison of serum amyloid A in horses with infectious and noninfectious respiratory diseases. J Equine Vet Sci 2017; 49:11–3.

31. Hooijberg EH, van den Hoven R, Tichy A, et al. Diagnostic and predictive capa-bility of routine laboratory tests for the diagnosis and staging of equine inflamma-tory disease. J Vet Intern Med 2014;28(5):1587–93.

32. Belgrave RL, Dickey MM, Arheart KL, et al. Assessment of serum amyloid A testing of horses and its clinical application in a specialized equine practice. J Am Vet Med Assoc 2013;243(1):113–9.

33. Stoneham SJ, Palmer L, Cash R, et al. Measurement of serum amyloid A in the neonatal foal using a latex agglutination immunoturbidimetric assay: determina-tion of the normal range, variation with age and response to disease. Equine Vet J 2001;33(6):599–603.

34. Pollock PJ, Prendergast M, Schumacher J, et al. Effects of surgery on the acute phase response in clinically normal and diseased horses. Vet Rec 2005;156(17): 538–42.

35. Hultén C, Demmers S. Serum amyloid A (SAA) as an aid in the management of infectious disease in the foal: comparison with total leucocyte count, neutrophil count and fibrinogen. Equine Vet J 2002;34(7):693–8.

36. Paltrinieri S, Giordano A, Villani M, et al. Influence of age and foaling on plasma protein electrophoresis and serum amyloid A and their possible role as markers of equine neonatal septicaemia. Vet J 2008;176(3):393–6.

37. Giguère S, Berghaus LJ, Miller CD. Clinical assessment of a point-of-care serum amyloid A assay in foals with bronchopneumonia. J Vet Intern Med 2016;30(4): 1338.

38. Gardner RB, Nydam DV, Luna JA, et al. Serum opsonization capacity, phagocy-tosis, and oxidative burst activity in neonatal foals in the intensive care unit. J Vet Intern Med 2007;21(4):797–805.

39. Duggan VE, Holyoak GR, MacAllister CG, et al. Amyloid A in equine colostrum and early milk. Vet Immunol Immunopathol 2008;121(1):150–5.

40. Hemberg E, Einarsson S, Kútvölgyi G, et al. Occurrence of bacteria and polymor-phonuclear leukocytes in fetal compartments at parturition; relationships with foal and mare health in the peripartum period. Theriogenology 2015;84(1):163–9.

41. Vandenplas ML, Moore JN, Barton MH, et al. Concentrations of serum amyloid A and lipopolysaccharide-binding protein in horses with colic. Am J Vet Res 2005; 66(9):1509–16.

42. Pihl TH, Scheepers E, Sanz M, et al. Acute-phase proteins as diagnostic markers in horses with colic. J Vet Emerg Crit Care (San Antonio) 2016;26(5):664–74.

43. Westerman TL, Foster CM, Tornquist SJ, et al. Evaluation of serum amyloid A and haptoglobin concentrations as prognostic indicators for horses with colic. J Am Vet Med Assoc 2016;248(8):935–40.

44. Dondi F, Lukacs RM, Gentilini F, et al. Serum amyloid A, haptoglobin, and ferritin in horses with colic: association with common clinicopathological variables and short-term outcome. Vet J 2015;205(1):50–5.

45. Copas VEN, Durham AE, Stratford CH, et al. In equine grass sickness, serum amyloid A and fibrinogen are elevated, and can aid differential diagnosis from non-inflammatory causes of colic. Vet Rec 2013;172(15):395.

46. Pihl TH, Andersen PH, Kjelgaard-Hansen M, et al. Serum amyloid A and haptoglobin concentrations in serum and peritoneal fluid of healthy horses and horses with acute abdominal pain. Vet Clin Pathol 2013;42(2):177–83.

47. Pihl TH, Scheepers E, Sanz M, et al. Influence of disease process and duration on acute phase proteins in serum and peritoneal fluid of horses with colic. J Vet Intern Med 2015;29(2):651–8.

48. Daniel AJ, Leise BS, Burgess BA, et al. Concentrations of serum amyloid A and plasma fibrinogen in horses undergoing emergency abdominal surgery. J Vet Emerg Crit Care (San Antonio) 2016;26(3):344–51.

49. Aitken MR, Stefanovski D, Southwood LL. Serum amyloid A concentration in postoperative colic horses and its association with postoperative complications. Vet Surg 2019;48(2):143–51.

50. De Cozar M, Sherlock C, Knowles E, et al. Serum amyloid A and plasma fibrinogen concentrations in horses following emergency exploratory celiotomy. Equine Vet J 2019;52(1):59–66.

51. Jacobsen S, Nielsen JV, Kjelgaard-Hansen M, et al. Acute phase response to surgery of varying intensity in horses: a preliminary study. Vet Surg 2009;38(6):762–9.

52. Endo Y, Tsuchiya T, Omura T, et al. Effects of pre-shipping marbofloxacin administration on fever and blood properties in healthy Thoroughbreds transported a long distance. J Vet Med Sci 2015;77(1):75–9.

53. Tsuchiya T, Hobo S, Endo Y, et al. Effects of a single dose of enrofloxacin on body temperature and tracheobronchial neutrophil count in healthy Thoroughbreds premedicated with interferon-α and undergoing long-distance transportation. Am J Vet Res 2012;73(7):968–72.

54. Casella S, Fazio F, Giannetto C, et al. Influence of transportation on serum concentrations of acute phase proteins in horse. Res Vet Sci 2012;93(2):914–7.

55. Hultén C, Sandgren B, Skiöldebrand E, et al. The acute phase protein serum amyloid A (SAA) as an inflammatory marker in equine influenza virus infection. Acta Vet Scand 1999;40(4):323–33.

56. Barton AK, Wirth C, Bondzio A, et al. Are pulmonary hemostasis and fibrinolysis out of balance in equine chronic pneumopathies? J Vet Sci 2017;18(3):349.

57. Leclere M, Lavoie-Lamoureux A, Lavoie J-P. Acute phase proteins in racehorses with inflammatory airway disease. J Vet Intern Med 2015;29(3):940–5.

58. Cohen ND, Chaffin MK, Vandenplas ML, et al. Study of serum amyloid A concentrations as a means of achieving early diagnosis of *Rhodococcus equi* pneumonia. Equine Vet J 2005;37(3):212–6.

59. Passamonti F, Vardi DM, Stefanetti V, et al. *Rhodococcus equi* pneumonia in foals: an assessment of the early diagnostic value of serum amyloid A and plasma fibrinogen concentrations in equine clinical practice. Vet J 2015;203(2):211–8.

60. Jacobsen S, Jensen JC, Frei S, et al. Use of serum amyloid A and other acute phase reactants to monitor the inflammatory response after castration in horses: a field study. Equine Vet J 2005;37(6):552–6.

61. Busk P, Jacobsen S, Martinussen T. Administration of perioperative penicillin reduces postoperative serum amyloid A response in horses being castrated standing. Vet Surg 2010;39(5):638–43.

62. Krakowski L, Bartoszek P, Krakowska I, et al. Serum amyloid A protein (SAA), haptoglobin (Hp) and selected hematological and biochemical parameters in wild mares before and after parturition. Pol J Vet Sci 2017;20(2):299–305.

63. Canisso IF, Ball BA, Cray C, et al. Serum amyloid A and haptoglobin concentrations are increased in plasma of mares with ascending placentitis in the absence of changes in peripheral leukocyte counts or fibrinogen concentration. Am J Reprod Immunol 2014;72(4):376–85.

64. Nash DM, Sheldon IM, Herath S, et al. Markers of the uterine innate immune response of the mare. Anim Reprod Sci 2010;119(1):31–9.

65. Christoffersen M, Woodward E, Bojesen AM, et al. Inflammatory responses to induced infectious endometritis in mares resistant or susceptible to persistent endometritis. BMC Vet Res 2012;8:41.

66. Mette C, Camilla Dooleweerdt B, Stine J, et al. Evaluation of the systemic acute phase response and endometrial gene expression of serum amyloid A and pro- and anti-inflammatory cytokines in mares with experimentally induced endometritis. Vet Immunol Immunopathol 2010;138(1):95–105.

67. Erol E, Jackson C, Horohov D, et al. Elevated serum amyloid A levels in cases of aborted equine fetuses due to fetal and placental infections. Theriogenology 2016;86(4):971–5.

68. Jacobsen S, Niewold TA, Halling-Thomsen M, et al. Serum amyloid A isoforms in serum and synovial fluid in horses with lipopolysaccharide-induced arthritis. Vet Immunol Immunopathol 2006;110(3–4):325–30.

69. Sanchez Teran AF, Rubio-Martinez LM, Villarino NF, et al. Effects of repeated intra-articular administration of amikacin on serum amyloid A, total protein and nucleated cell count in synovial fluid from healthy horses. Equine Vet J Suppl 2012;(43):12–6.

70. Sanchez-Teran AF, Bracamonte JL, Hendrick S, et al. Effect of arthroscopic lavage on systemic and synovial fluid serum amyloid A in healthy horses. Vet Surg 2016;45(2):223–30.

71. Sanchez-Teran AF, Bracamonte JL, Hendrick S, et al. Effect of repeated through-and-through joint lavage on serum amyloid A in synovial fluid from healthy horses. Vet J 2016;210:30–3.

72. Jacobsen S, Thomsen MH, Nanni S. Concentrations of serum amyloid A in serum and synovial fluid from healthy horses and horses with joint disease. Am J Vet Res 2006;67(10):1738–42.

73. Robinson CS, Singer ER, Piviani M, et al. Are serum amyloid A or D-lactate useful to diagnose synovial contamination or sepsis in horses? Vet Rec 2017; 181(16):425.

74. Ludwig EK, Brandon Wiese R, Graham MR, et al. Serum and synovial fluid serum amyloid A response in equine models of synovitis and septic arthritis. Vet Surg 2016;45(7):859–67.

75. Haltmayer E, Schwendenwein I, Licka TF. Course of serum amyloid A (SAA) plasma concentrations in horses undergoing surgery for injuries penetrating synovial structures, an observational clinical study. BMC Vet Res 2017;13:137.

76. Menzies-Gow NJ, Wray H, Bailey SR, et al. The effect of exercise on plasma concentrations of inflammatory markers in normal and previously laminitic ponies. Equine Vet J 2014;46(3):317–21.

77. Bamford NJ, Potter SJ, Baskerville CL, et al. Influence of dietary restriction and low-intensity exercise on weight loss and insulin sensitivity in obese equids. J Vet Intern Med 2019;33(1):280–6.

78. Suagee JK, Corl BA, Crisman MV, et al. Relationships between body condition score and plasma inflammatory cytokines, insulin, and lipids in a mixed population of light-breed horses. J Vet Intern Med 2013;27(1):157–63.

79. Cywinska A, Witkowski L, Szarska E, et al. Serum amyloid A (SAA) concentration after training sessions in Arabian race and endurance horses. BMC Vet Res 2013; 9(1):91.

80. Cywińska A, Szarska E, Górecka R, et al. Acute phase protein concentrations after limited distance and long distance endurance rides in horses. Res Vet Sci 2012;93(3):1402–6.

81. Kristensen L, Buhl R, Nostell K, et al. Acute exercise does not induce an acute phase response (APR) in Standardbred trotters. Can J Vet Res 2014;78(2): 97–102.

82. Mack SJ, Kirkby K, Malalana F, et al. Elevations in serum muscle enzyme activities in racehorses due to unaccustomed exercise and training. Vet Rec 2014; 174(6):145.

83. Andersen UV, Reinemeyer CR, Toft N, et al. Physiologic and systemic acute phase inflammatory responses in young horses repeatedly infected with cyathostomins and Strongylus vulgaris. Vet Parasitol 2014;201(1–2):67–74.

84. Nielsen MK, Betancourt A, Lyons ET, et al. Characterization of the inflammatory response to anthelmintic treatment of ponies with cyathostominosis. Vet J 2013; 198(2):457–62.

85. Nielsen MK, Loynachan AT, Jacobsen S, et al. Local and systemic inflammatory and immunologic reactions to cyathostomin larvicidal therapy in horses. Vet Immunol Immunopathol 2015;168(3–4):203–10.

86. Andersen SA, Petersen HH, Ersbøll AK, et al. Vaccination elicits a prominent acute phase response in horses. Vet J 2012;191(2):199–202.

87. Labelle AL, Hamor RE, Macneill AL, et al. Effects of ophthalmic disease on concentrations of plasma fibrinogen and serum amyloid A in the horse. Equine Vet J 2011;43(4):460–5.

88. Mittelman NS, Stefanovski D, Johnson AL. Utility of C-reactive protein and serum amyloid A in the diagnosis of equine protozoal myeloencephalitis. J Vet Intern Med 2018;32(5):1726–30.

Point-of-Care Diagnostics in Equine Practice

Nathan M. Slovis, DVM, CHT*, Nimet Browne, DVM, MPH,
Rana Bozorgmanesh, BVetMed

KEYWORDS

- Point of care • Polymerase chain reaction • Serum amyloid A • L-Lactate
- Cardiac troponin I • Immunoglobulin G

KEY POINTS

- Advantages of Point of Care Diagnostics for the equine practitioner would be to treat faster with test results while reducing the initial guess work and offering the patient optimal care with the end goal of better clinical outcomes.
- In the last two decades the diversity of tests that can be performed using POCT devices has expanded considerably.
- Recent advances in diagnostic technology have allowed for the development of various Equine Point of Care diagnostics.

Point-of-care testing (POCT) refers to benchtop diagnostic modalities that have been translated into portable and easy-to-use formats suitable for patient-side use. Recent advances in diagnostic technology have allowed the development of a growing collection of POCT assays available to equine practitioners. Advantages include rapid results that reduce initial guesswork and promote diagnosis-targeted patient care, which may ultimately provide better clinical outcomes. Small handheld devices comprise most POCT technologies, providing qualitative or quantitative determination of an increasing range of analytes, including critical care analyzers and, more recently, hematology and immunology analyzers. New emerging devices include those using molecular techniques such as the polymerase chain reaction to provide infectious disease testing in a POCT format. Commercially available equine POCT are discussed in this article, highlighting some of the latest versions of these technologies.

Point-of-care diagnostics refers to benchtop diagnostic modalities that have been translated into portable and easy-to-use formats suitable for patient-side use. The volume of human POCT has steadily increased over the 40 years since its introduction. That growth is likely to continue, driven by changes in health care designed to deliver less costly care closer to the patients' homes.[1] Small handheld devices comprise

Hagyard Equine Medical Institute, McGee Medical Center, 4250 Iron Works Pike, Lexington, KY 40511, USA
* Corresponding author.
E-mail address: nslovis@hagyard.com

Vet Clin Equine 36 (2020) 161–171
https://doi.org/10.1016/j.cveq.2019.12.007
0749-0739/20/© 2020 Elsevier Inc. All rights reserved.

most POCT technologies, providing qualitative or quantitative determination of an increasing range of analytes. Also included in POCT are versions of traditional bench-top devices that have been reduced in size and complexity. These devices include critical care analyzers and, more recently, hematology and immunology analyzers. New emerging devices include those using molecular techniques such as polymerase chain reaction (PCR) to provide infectious disease testing in a POCT format. The World Health Organization (WHO) has provided guidelines for those developing POCT devices (**Box 1**).[1]

Recent advances in diagnostic technology have allowed the development of a growing collection of equine POCT. Advantages of POCT for equine practitioners include rapid results that reduce initial guesswork, promotion of diagnosis-targeted patient care, and potentially better clinical outcomes (**Fig. 1**). Commercially available POCT for horses is discussed later, highlighting features of the latest versions of these technologies.

CLINICAL PATHOLOGY

A myriad of handheld devices exist for equine POCT, ranging from simple dipstick indicators to sophisticated, cartridge-based devices used for blood gas analysis.

Blood Gas Analysis

Multiple handheld analyzers are available for equine blood gas analyses. The IRMA Trupoint Blood Analysis System (LifeHealth, Roseville, MN) and i-STAT are used commonly for this purpose. Compared with traditional laboratory analyzers, the i-STAT was found to be reliable for blood gas analysis in equine venous blood samples.[2,3] The i-STAT is temperature dependent and contains a built-in thermostat that restricts its use outside of optimum operating temperatures. Cartridges must be refrigerated. The older i-STAT models are currently being superseded by the newer i-STAT 1. Other available handheld blood gas analyzers include the Heska Element POC, which displays results within 35 seconds and does not require refrigeration of the test card; Enterprise POC (EPOC) (Alere, Waltham, MA), VetStat analyzer (IDEXX Laboratories, Westbrook, ME) and StatPal II (Unifet, Inc, La Jolla, CA). One study showed acceptable agreement between the EPOC and a NOVA benchtop analyzer (NOVA, NOVA Biomedical, Waltham, MA) in 75 samples from

---

Box 1
The ASSURED guidelines (recommended by World Health Organization) that indicate the features that should be designed into all point-of-care testing devices

- Affordable: for those at risk of infection
- Sensitive: minimal false-negatives
- Specific: minimal false-positives
- User friendly: minimal steps to perform test
- Rapid and robust: short turnaround time and no need for refrigerated storage
- Equipment free: no complex equipment
- Delivered: to end users

From St John A, Price CP. Existing and Emerging Technologies for Point-of-Care Testing. *Clin Biochem Rev.* 2014;35(3):155-167; with permission.

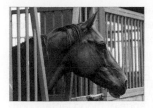

**RESULTS IN
30 MIN**

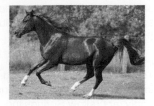

**UP TO 3 D
OF WAITING FOR
CENTRALIZED
LABORATORIES**

**During the waiting period, care
must continue, this leads to:**

- Initial guess work for infections
- Incorrect patient treatment
- Transmission of disease from an
  infected patient

Give immediate & optimal care to:

- Realize better patient outcomes
- Initiate outbreak management
  protocol immediately
- Have happier patients and owners
- Save costs for all parties

Fig. 1. POCT.

42 horses, except for partial pressure of carbon dioxide (Pco_2) and chloride.[4] Another study in 100 horses showed that performance (including precision and agreement) of EPOC versus Radiometer ABL77 benchtop analyzer was good for some tests, such as pH, oxygen tension, potassium, bicarbonate, and oxygen saturation of hemoglobin, but not for others, including Pco_2 and ionized calcium.[5] In a study comparing the EPOC and VetStat with a Cobas benchtop analyzer in 41 venous blood samples from 23 horses, the VetStat yielded reliable results for pH, Pco_2, potassium, and bicarbonate. However, sodium, chloride, and oxygen tension results were less reliable. The EPOC analyzer achieved acceptable results for potassium and bicarbonate, whereas results for pH, Pco_2, oxygen tension, and sodium were considered less accurate.[6] The StatPal II has shown acceptable precision for measurement of blood gas analytes in equine blood.[7] Although there were significant differences between results for some analytes comparing the StatPal II with benchtop analyzers (Instrumentation Laboratory, IL series, in 27 samples and Radiometer, ABL series, in 78 samples), the investigators considered these changes to be clinically irrelevant. However, users should remain aware of the differences and not use analyzers interchangeably.[8]

L-Lactate

Measuring blood and/or peritoneal fluid L-lactate concentration is an established practice in the diagnostic evaluation and management of sick equine patients. Heparinized plasma and whole blood samples are not interchangeable because the lactate distribution between red blood cells and plasma varies unevenly during and after exercise, particularly in horses.[9,10] Whole blood or peritoneal fluid samples should be run within

30 minutes of collection because lactate concentrations may increase during storage.[9] Although peritoneal fluid may be centrifuged before measurement of lactate, this is not required.[5]

i-STAT (Abaxis)

The i-STAT measures blood lactate as a panel including other blood gas tests. In 1 study, there was a significant bias noted between the i-STAT and automated lactate analyzer (Yellow Springs Inc, Yellow Springs, OH) over the range of blood lactate concentrations evaluated (0.5–18.0 mmol/L); however, the lactate result was highly reproducible.[11] The i-STAT also has a built-in thermostat that prevents function when out of the optimum operating temperature range (16°–30°C).[11] Lactate may also be performed, measured in synovial fluid, yielding acceptable results to the Radiometer ABL benchtop analyzers (Radiometer, ABL series).[12]

Accutrend (formerly Accusport) (Roche Diagnostics, Mannheim, Germany)

This handheld portable analyzer uses an enzymatic colorimetric method and has plasma and blood modes. Close agreement was shown between the Accutrend and a NOVA benchtop blood gas analyzer (NOVA, NOVA Biomedical, Waltham, MA) when lactate concentrations were measured in plasma. Results were less consistent at higher lactate concentrations but reliable enough to show trends. Although whole blood may be used with this analyzer to identify clinically important hyperlactatemia, results are likely not reliable enough to monitor trends with sequential monitoring.[13] Similarly, other studies evaluating the Accutrend have found that the device greatly underestimated the blood lactate concentration at concentrations greater than 10 mmol/L. A similar underestimation occurred when the packed cell volume was greater than 53%. However, these studies found, in contrast with blood, that plasma lactate concentration was in the range of 0.8 to 20 mmol/L.[14–17]

Lactate Pro (Arkray Global Business, Kyoto, Japan)

The Lactate Pro has recently been superseded by the Lactate Pro 2. A linear relationship in blood lactate concentration was shown between the Lactate Pro and a Radiometer benchtop analyzer, with good correlation between the analyzers ($r = 0.90$) over a range of lactate concentrations of 1.0 to 18.6 mmol/L. The repeatability for the Lactate Pro was also high.[18] Compared with the Lactate Plus and Lactate Scout, the Lactate Pro had the highest level of agreement with a chromogenic benchtop assay for lactate measurement in peritoneal fluid. Contrasting with the previous study,[18] the intra-analyzer variability was high for the Lactate Pro (15% coefficient of variation [CV]) at medium blood lactate concentrations (3–7 mmol/L).[19]

Lactate Scout (SensLab GmbH, Leipzig, Germany)

The Lactate Scout requires 0.5 μL of whole blood and gives a reading in 10 seconds. When 3 portable lactate analyzers were compared, the Lactate Scout had high intra-analyzer variability at medium blood lactate concentrations (17% CV). Lactate measurements in blood and peritoneal fluid were more in agreement with the chromogenic benchtop analyzer at low (<3 mmol/L) versus high (>7 mmol/L) lactate concentrations.[19]

Lactate Plus (Nova Biomedical, Waltham, Massachusetts)

The Lactate Plus uses 0.7 μL of whole blood to measure the lactate concentration in 13 seconds. Although the device significantly underestimates blood lactate concentrations by 0.39 mmol/L compared with a chromogenic benchtop analyzer (Lactate kit 737–10, Trinity Biotech, Jamestown, NY), it was considered reliable for monitoring blood lactate concentrations in horses on a conditioning program. The latter conclusion was based on a good correlation ($r = 0.978$) between the Lactate Plus and the benchtop analyzer and results from difference or Bland-Altman plots.[20]

Hematology and Chemistry

Some hematologic and biochemical tests can also be performed stall-side using the Abaxis i-STAT and other POCT instruments, as mentioned earlier. Caution should be used when interpreting hematocrit (HCT) from the i-STAT (results may be falsely low)[2,3] and EPOC, as indicated earlier. The Heska Element provides results for several biochemical analytes (electrolytes, urea nitrogen, creatinine, and glucose), as well as the blood gas tests previously mentioned. Comparison with benchtop analyzers has not been reported for blood analysis in horses.

Cardiac Troponin I

Cardiac troponin I (cTnI) is a sensitive and specific biomarker of myocardial injury. The i-STAT can measure cTnI in 16 to 22 μL of plasma, serum, or heparinized whole blood within 10 minutes. It uses a 2-site enzyme-linked immunosorbent assay (ELISA) with 2 monoclonal antibodies raised against different epitopes of human cTnI and, per the manufacturer, has an analytical sensitivity of 0.02 ng/mL and a reportable range of 0.0 to 50 ng/mL. Normal cTnI concentrations for adult horses with the i-STAT are 0.00 to 0.06 ng/mL. In horses with and without experimentally induced cardiac disease, the i-STAT and benchtop immunoassay (ACCESS Immunoassay, Ohio State University Medical Center Reference Laboratory, Columbus, OH) provided similar results for plasma cTnI.[21] However, the authors have encountered multiple error messages when attempting to use the i-STAT to measure cTnI concentrations in neonatal foals.

Serum Amyloid A

Tissue injury resulting from trauma, infection, neoplasia, or inflammation results in a highly complex set of innate immune reactions, known as the acute phase response (APR).[22] In addition to activation and release of inflammatory molecules and cytokines, the APR is responsible for increased hepatic synthesis and release of acute phase proteins (APPs).[22] Serum amyloid A (SAA) is a small apoprotein that circulates with high-density lipoproteins.[22,23] The protein is degraded in the liver and has a half-life of 30 minutes to 2 hours.[22,24] SAA has been studied extensively as a marker of inflammation in the horse because it has many characteristics that make it uniquely suitable as a diagnostic test. These properties include a low basal concentration followed by a rapid, profound increase with the onset of an APR. In addition, changes in this APP seems to correlate with the degree of tissue damage, and concentrations decrease or increase with recovery or development of secondary infections, respectively.[22,25–27] Plasma concentrations of SAA in healthy horses range from 0.5 to 20 mg/L, although reference intervals in neonates and older horses may be slightly higher.[22,28,29] SAA has also been evaluated as a tool to evaluate fitness and the APR after exercise (for more information, please refer to the article on SAA in this issue).

There are several methods for measuring and quantifying SAA in horses, including single radial immunodiffusion, ELISA, slide reversed passive agglutination, electroimmunoassay, and immunoturbidometry.[29–33] The current POCT analyzer is a proprietary lateral flow, membrane-based immunoassay (StableLab EQ handheld reader with SAA test and pipette pack) that is available as semiquantitative and quantitative versions. The POCT analyzer showed fair agreement with an automated analyzer-based turbidimetric immunoassay ($r = 0.86$, with some outliers having much higher or lower concentrations on a difference plot) but had high intra-assay and intra-assay variability (13%–18% and 14%–46%, respectively) in serum or plasma. Blood SAA concentrations showed a consistent negative bias (POCT analyzer reading lower than serum/plasma results with the automated analyzer) at SAA concentrations greater than 500 ng/L.[22,33,34] The HCT did not affect test results in whole blood (based on a lack of correlation between the HCT and SAA concentrations; $r^2 = 0.006$). In addition, there was high interbatch variability for results greater than 1000 mg/L, as seen in horses with severe, acute inflammation, which may preclude serial monitoring in such horses.[34] The results of the latter study indicate that the POCT analyzer can provide useful information regarding SAA concentration in serum or plasma of horses when values are less than 500 mg/L.[34] Despite the POCT device being designed for use with whole blood, results in whole blood are less accurate and should be expected to be lower than in serum/plasma; therefore, when serial monitoring is used, the same sample type should be used.[34]

Immunoglobulin G

One of the most widely used POCT assays available for horses is the stall-side immunoglobulin (Ig) G test. Traditionally, the single radial immunodiffusion (RID) was considered to be the most accurate test for quantitative measurement of antibody levels in foals; however, testing must be performed in a laboratory and results typically take up to 24 hours from time of receipt.[35–37] As a result, numerous stall-side diagnostic tests have been developed. These tests include the glutaraldehyde coagulation test (GammaCheck-E), zinc sulfate turbidity test (Equi-Z), latex agglutination test (Foalcheck), enzyme immunoassay (SNAP test), and a new turbidimetric immunoassay (ARS Foal IgG Test). The SNAP test is a semiquantitative enzyme immunoassay that provides quick, reliable, stall-side results.[36–38] In comparison, the more recently available turbidimetric immunoassay has also been shown to provide fast, reliable results.[35,37,39] The RID method has been supplanted by an automated immunoturbidometric assay in most laboratories and this also has a fast turnaround time.[40]

PATHOGEN DETECTION

Pathogen detection in POCT assays is usually based on immunologic-based or PCR-based techniques. Several PCR-based POCT systems have recently entered the veterinary market for infectious disease testing. Companies such as Fluxergy LLC (Irvine, CA), Horiba's POCKIT Central PCR System (Japan), and Credo Biomedical's QubeMDx (Singapore) offer a variety of veterinary PCR assays; however, Credo Biomedical only offers canine and feline testing at this time. These PCR POCT systems can deliver results in as little as 15 minutes, with most averaging between 45 and 60 minutes.

Streptococcus equi

Fluxergy have recently completed a developed of PCR-based POCT for the detection of *Streptococcus equi* subspecies *equi*, the causative agent of strangles. The reaction is based on detection of the eqbE gene of *S equi*, and testing can be done on nasal secretions, respiratory lavages, and pus. Testing done at the University of California Davis showed an overall sensitivity of 89% compared with quantitative PCR (qPCR) for *S equi*, with sensitivity depending on bacterial load as determined by cycle threshold with qPCR (ie, how many amplification cycles it takes to detect the DNA in the sample). For strongly and moderately positive bacterial loads (arbitrarily defined as computed tomography [CT] values <32 and CT values 32–35, respectively), the

POCT analyzer had a 100% agreement with qPCR, whereas a weak bacterial load (arbitrarily defined CT values >35) had 71% agreement with qPCR. The reported specificity was 100% when testing samples containing *Streptococcus zooepidemicus* or those lacking bacteria. The analytical sensitivity of the POCT analyzer was 277 eqbE gene copies (Dr Nicola Pusterla, personal communication, 2019).

Borrelia burgdorferi and Anaplasma phagocytophilum

Historically, confirmation of *Borrelia burgdorferi* infection in horses has required either laboratory-based ELISA or immunoblotting assays (Western blot), taking hours to days to obtain results. The POCT SNAP4DX ELISA evaluates for the presence of the synthetic peptide C6 derived from the IR6 region within the *B burgdorferi* membrane protein VlsE, as well as peptides derived from the immunodominant p44 protein of *Anaplasma phagocytophilum*. The test also performs antigen testing for *Dirofilaria immitis* and *Ehrlichia canis*.[41–43] The SNAP4DX ELISA was first evaluated using serum from ponies experimentally infected with *B burgdorferi*. Results indicated high specificity (100%) with poor sensitivity (63%), indicating that it may be useful as a screening tool for Lyme borreliosis in horses in endemic areas.[42,43] However, even in such areas, the test may yield false-negative results. With respect to *A phagocytophilum*, the SNAP4DX ELISA had 100% sensitivity and specificity compared with an immunofluorescent assay.[44] However, when used to evaluate seroprevalence of disease in a non-endemic area (0.5%–0.7% prevalence), the test showed very low sensitivity (7.4%) compared with an indirect immunofluorescent assay, indicating that the test should be used with caution in a low-prevalence setting.[45]

Rotavirus

Rotaviruses are double-stranded, nonenveloped RNA viruses. Rotavirus is subdivided into several groups (A through G) based on differences in the group-specific inner capsid protein, VP6. There are 3 rotavirus groups (A, B, and C) that cause disease in humans, compared with only 1 group that affects horses (group A).[46] Because equine rotavirus is among the group A strains, it would be anticipated that test kits marketed for human use that are based on antibodies directed against the core protein VP6 (antigenically conserved among group A rotavirus strains) should detect the virus in equine feces. These test kits are anecdotally being used as a quick equine POCT assay for rotavirus detection in many equine hospitals, because they yield results within 10 minutes. However, in a recent study done by one of the authors (N.M.S.), 1 of these kits (Immunocard Stat, Meridian Biosecience Inc, Cincinnati, OH) yielded false-negative results compared with an equine-specific real-time PCR assay (IDEXX Equine Diarrhea Panel RealPCR). Thus, practitioners must remember that these kits require validation before anticipating they will yield accurate results.

Fecal Egg Count

The fecal egg count is traditionally performed by weighing a certain amount of feces, homogenizing it by mixing, and then separating parasite eggs from debris by flotation. The fecal egg count is then quantified using a McMaster counting chamber. Although performed routinely, the process can be laborious and open to human error.[47–49] Other homogenization techniques have been developed to make parasite quantification easier and less labor intensive, such as the Flotac and Mini-Flotac systems (Veterinary Parasitology and Parasitic Diseases Department of Veterinary Medicine and Animal Productions University of Naples Federico II). The later techniques have been designed to accommodate a larger volume of fecal suspension, leading to a lower limit of detection.[50] The Mini-Flotac system is potentially a stall-side device, because it does not require a centrifuge, just a microscope. The Mini-Flotac is composed of two 1-mL flotation chambers within a device containing a base, a reading disc (required 40× objective), and a translational disc. It is used with a 5-g Fill-Flotac system for generating a homogenized filtered sample, which can then be loaded directly into the counting chambers. Egg counts are then performed routinely with a microscope. A smartphone-based application has been developed to reduce operator error in microscope quantification (The Parasight System, MEP Equine Solutions, Lexington, KY).[47,48,51–53] This application is based on detection of fluorescently labeled eggs in the McMaster counting chamber and requires a fluorescent imaging device (smartphone application) or microscope as well as harvesting stained eggs off a 27-μum filter.[47,48,53] The smartphone counting methods had higher precision than the standard McMaster or Mini-Flotac techniques and similar accuracy to the McMaster chamber. Accuracies for the smartphone application and the McMaster chamber were lower than for the Mini-Flotac method.

DISCLOSURE

The authors have nothing to declare.

REFERENCES

1. St John A, Price CP. Existing and emerging technologies for point-of-care testing. Clin Biochem Rev 2014;35(3):155–67.
2. Looney AL, Ludders J, Erb HN, et al. Use of a handheld device for analysis of blood electrolyte concentrations and blood gas partial pressures in dogs and horses. J Am Vet Med Assoc 1998;213(4):526–30.
3. Peiró JR, Borges AS, Gonçalves RC, et al. Evaluation of a portable clinical analyzer for the determination of blood gas partial pressures, electrolyte concentrations, and hematocrit in venous blood samples collected from cattle, horses, and sheep. Am J Vet Res 2010;71(5):515–21.
4. Elmeshreghi TN, Grubb TL, Greene SA, et al. Comparison of enterprise point-of-care and nova biomedical critical care xpress analyzers for determination of arterial pH, blood gas, and electrolyte values in canine and equine blood. Vet Clin Pathol 2018;47(3):415–24.
5. Bardell D, West E, Mark Senior J. Evaluation of a new handheld point-of-care blood gas analyser using 100 equine blood samples. Vet Anaesth Analg 2017; 44(1):77–85.
6. Kirsch K, Detilleux J, Serteyn D, et al. Comparison of two portable clinical analyzers to one stationary analyzer for the determination of blood gas partial pressures and blood electrolyte concentrations in horses. PLoS One 2019;14(2). https://doi.org/10.1371/journal.pone.0211104.
7. Klein LV, Soma LR, Nann LE. Accuracy and precision of the portable StatPal II and the laboratory-based NOVA stat profile 1 for measurement of pH, Pco2, and Po2 in equine blood. Vet Surg 1999;28(1):67–76.
8. Mitten LA, Hinchcliff KW, Sams R. A portable blood gas analyzer for equine venous blood. J Vet Intern Med 1995;9(5):353–6.
9. Biedler A, Schneider S, Bach F, et al. Methodological aspects of lactate measurement - evaluation of the accuracy of photometric and biosensor methods. Open Anesthesiol J 2007;1(1):1–5.
10. Rainger JE, Evans DL, Hodgson DR, et al. Distribution of lactate in plasma anderythrocytes during and after exercise in horses. Br Vet J 1995;151(3):299–310.

11. Silverman SC, Birks EK. Evaluation of the i-STAT hand-held chemical analyser during treadmill and endurance exercise. Equine Vet J Suppl 2002;34:551–4.
12. Dechant JE, Symm WA, Nieto JE. Comparison of pH, lactate, and glucose analysis of equine synovial fluid using a portable clinical analyzer with a bench-top blood gas analyzer. Vet Surg 2011;40(7):811–6.
13. Tennent-Brown BS, Wilkins PA, Lindborg S, et al. Assessment of a point-of-care lactate monitor in emergency admissions of adult horses to a referral hospital. J Vet Intern Med 2007;21(5):1090–8.
14. Evans DL, Golland LC. Accuracy of accusport for measurement of lactate concentrations in equine blood and plasma. Equine Vet J 1996. https://doi.org/10.1111/j.2042-3306.1996.tb03111.x.
15. Constable P, Sulimai N, Tinkler S, et al. Accuracy of a point-of-care lactate analyzer for measuring blood and Plasma L-Lactate concentrations in exercising Standardbreds. Equine Vet J 2014;46(S46):20.
16. Lindner A. Measurement of plasma lactate concentration with accusport. Equine Vet J 1996;28(5):403–5.
17. Schulman ML, Nurton JP, Guthrie AJ. Use of the Accusport semi-automated analyser to determine blood lactate as an aid in the clinical assessment of horses with colic. J S Afr Vet Assoc 2001;28(5):398–402.
18. Van Oldruitenborgh-Oosterbaan MMS, Van Den Broek ETW, Spierenburg AJ. Evaluation of the usefulness of the portable device Lactate Pro for measurement of lactate concentrations in equine whole blood. J Vet Diagn Investig 2008; 20(1):83–5.
19. Nieto JE, Dechant JE, le Jeune SS, et al. Evaluation of 3 handheld portable analyzers for measurement of L-Lactate concentrations in blood and peritoneal fluid of horses with colic. Vet Surg 2015;44(3):366–72.
20. Hauss AA, Stablein CK, Fisher AL, et al. Validation of the lactate plus lactate meter in the horse and its use in a conditioning program. J Equine Vet Sci 2014; 34(9):1064–8.
21. Kraus MS, Jesty SA, Gelzer AR, et al. Measurement of plasma cardiac troponin I concentration by use of a point-of-care analyzer in clinically normal horses and horses with experimentally induced cardiac disease. Am J Vet Res 2010; 71(1):55–9.
22. Jacobsen S, Andersen PH. The acute phase protein serum amyloid a (SAA) as a marker of inflammation in horses. Equine Vet Educ 2007;19(1):38–46.
23. Sletten K, Husebekk A, Husby G. The primary structure of equine Serum Amyloid A (SAA) protein. Scand J Immunol 1989;30(1):117–22.
24. Uhlar CM, Whitehead AS. Serum amyloid A, the major vertebrate acute-phase reactant. Eur J Biochem 1999;265(2):501–23.
25. Kent J. Acute phase proteins: their use in veterinary diagnosis. Br Vet J 1992; 148(4):279–82.
26. Crisman MV, Kent Scarratt W, Zimmerman KL. Blood proteins and inflammation in the horse. Vet Clin North Am Equine Pract 2008;24(2):285–97.
27. Aitken MR, Stefanovski D, Southwood LL. Serum amyloid A concentration in postoperative colic horses and its association with postoperative complications. Vet Surg 2019;48(2):143–51.
28. Jacobsen S, Kjelgaard-Hansen M. Evaluation of a commercially available apparatus for measuring the acute phase protein serum amyloid a in horses. Vet Rec 2008;163(11):327–30.
29. Nunokawa Y, Fujinaga T, Taira T, et al. Evaluation of Serum Amyloid A protein as an acute-phase reactive protein in horses. J Vet Med Sci 1993;55(6):1011–6.

30. Stoneham SJ, Palmer L, Cash R, et al. Measurement of serum amyloid A in the neonatal foal using a latex agglutination immunoturbidimetric assay: determination of the normal range, variation with age and response to disease. Equine Vet J 2010;33(6):599–603.

31. Wakimoto Y. Slide revered passive latex agglutination test: a simple, rapid and practical method for equine Serum Amyloid A (SAA) protein determination. Jpn J Vet Res 1996;44(1):43.

32. Chavatte PM, Pepys MB, Roberts B, et al. Measurement of serum amyloid A protein (SAA) as an aid to differential diagnosis of infection in newborn foals. In: Equine Infectious Diseases VI: Proceedings of the Sixth International Conference. July 7–11, 1991.

33. Jacobsen S, Kjelgaard-Hansen M, Hagbard Petersen H, et al. Evaluation of a commercially available human serum amyloid A (SAA) turbidometric immunoassay for determination of equine SAA concentrations. Vet J 2006;172(2):315–9.

34. Schwartz D, Pusterla N, Jacobsen S, et al. Analytical validation of a new point-of-care assay for serum amyloid A in horses. Equine Vet J 2018;50(5):678–83.

35. Ujvari S, Schwarzwald CC, Fouché N, et al. Validation of a point-of-care quantitative equine IgG Turbidimetric immunoassay and Comparison of IgG concentrations measured with radial immunodiffusion and a point-of-care IgG ELISA. J Vet Intern Med 2017;31(4):1170–7.

36. Metzger N, Hinchcliff KW, Hardy J, et al. Usefulness of a commercial equine IgG test and serum protein concentration as indicators of failure of transfer of passive immunity in hospitalized foals. J Vet Intern Med 2006. https://doi.org/10.1892/0891-6640(2006)20[382:UOACEI]2.0.CO;2.

37. Pusterla N, Pusterla JB, Spier SJ, et al. Evaluation of the SNAP foal IgG test for the semiquantitative measurement of immunoglobin G in foals. Vet Rec 2002;151(9):258–60.

38. Davis R, Giguère S. Evaluation of five commercially available assays and measurement of serum total protein concentration via refractometry for the diagnosis of failure of passive transfer of immunity in foals. J Am Vet Med Assoc 2005;227(10):1640–5.

39. Kent JE, Blackmore DJ. Measurement of IgG in equine blood by immunoturbidimetry and latex agglutination. Equine Vet J 1985;17(2):125–9.

40. Davis DG, Schaefer DMW, Hinchcliff KW, et al. Measurement of serum IgG in foals by radial immunodiffusion and automated turbidimetric immunoassay. J Vet Intern Med 2005. https://doi.org/10.1892/0891-6640(2005)19<93:MOSIIF>2.0.CO;2.

41. Schvartz G, Epp T, Burgess HJ, et al. Comparison between available serologic tests for detecting antibodies against Anaplasma phagocytophilum and Borrelia burgdorferi in horses in Canada. J Vet Diagn Investig 2015;27(4):540–6.

42. Johnson AL, Divers TJ, Chang YF. Validation of an in-clinic enzyme-linked immunosorbent assay kit for diagnosis of Borrelia burgdorferi infection in horses. J Vet Diagn Investig 2008;20(3):321–4.

43. Divers TJ, Gardner RB, Madigan JE, et al. Borrelia burgdorferi infection and lyme disease in North American horses: a consensus statement. J Vet Intern Med 2018;32(2):617–32.

44. Chandrashekar R, Daniluk D, Moffitt S, et al. Serologic diagnosis of equine borreliosis: evaluation of an in-clinic enzyme-linked immunosorbent assay (SNAP (R) 4Dx (R)). Int J Appl Res Vet Med 2008;6(3):145–50.

45. Schvartz G, Epp T, Burgess HJ, et al. Seroprevalence of equine granulocytic anaplasmosis and lyme borreliosis in Canada as determined by a point-of-care enzyme-linked immunosorbent assay (ELISA). Can Vet J 2015;56(6):575–80.

46. Estes MK, Cohen J. Rotavirus gene structure and function. Microbiol Rev 1989; 53(4):410–49.
47. Scare JA, Slusarewicz P, Noel ML, et al. Evaluation of accuracy and precision of a smartphone based automated parasite egg counting system in comparison to the McMaster and Mini-FLOTAC methods. Vet Parasitol 2017;247:85–92.
48. Noel ML, Scare JA, Bellaw JL, et al. Accuracy and precision of Mini-FLOTAC and McMaster techniques for determining equine Strongyle egg counts. J Equine Vet Sci 2017;48:182–7.
49. Vidyashankar AN, Kaplan RM, Chan S. Statistical approach to measure the efficacy of anthelmintic treatment on horse farms. Parasitology 2007;134(14): 2027–39.
50. Cringoli G, Maurelli MP, Levecke B, et al. The Mini-FLOTAC technique for the diagnosis of helminth and protozoan infections in humans and animals. Nat Protoc 2017;12(9):1723–32.
51. Ghazali KH, Hadi RS, Zeehaida M. Microscopy image processing analaysis for automatic detection of human intestinal parasites ALO and TTO. In: 2013 International Conference on Electronics, Computer and Computation, ICECCO 2013. November 7-9, 2013. https://doi.org/10.1109/ICECCO.2013.6718223.
52. Hadi RS, Ghazali KH, Khalidin IZ, et al. Human parasitic worm detection using image processing technique. In: ISCAIE 2012 - 2012 IEEE Symposium on Computer Applications and Industrial Electronics. December 3-4, 2012. https://doi.org/10.1109/ISCAIE.2012.6482095.
53. Slusarewicz P, Pagano S, Mills C, et al. Automated parasite faecal egg counting using fluorescence labelling, smartphone image capture and computational image analysis. Int J Parasitol 2016;46(8):485–93.

Printed and bound by CPI Group (UK) Ltd, Croydon, CR0 4YY

03/10/2024

01040408-0014